KILLER COLAS

KILLER COLAS

THE HARD TRUTH ABOUT SOFT DRINKS

NANCY APPLETON, PhD
G.N. JACOBS

SQUAREONE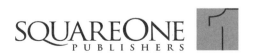
PUBLISHERS

COVER DESIGNER: Jeannie Tudor
EDITORS: Marie Caratozzolo and Michael Weatherhead
TYPESETTER: Gary A. Rosenberg

The information and advice contained in this book are based upon the research and the personal and professional experiences of the authors. They are not intended as a substitute for consulting with a healthcare professional. The publisher and author are not responsible for any adverse effects or consequences resulting from the use of any of the suggestions, preparations, or procedures discussed in this book. All matters pertaining to your physical health should be supervised by a healthcare professional. It is a sign of wisdom, not cowardice, to seek a second or third opinion.

Square One Publishers
115 Herricks Road
Garden City Park, NY 11040
(516) 535-2010 • (877) 900-BOOK
www.squareonepublishers.com

Library of Congress Cataloging-in-Publication Data
Appleton, Nancy.
  Killer colas : the hard truth about soft drinks / Nancy Appleton and G.N. Jacobs.
     p. cm.
  Includes bibliographical references and index.
  ISBN 978-0-7570-0341-7 (alk. paper)
  1. Carbonated beverages—Health aspects—Popular works. 2. Soft drinks—Popular works. I. Jacobs, G. N. II. Title.
  TP630.A67 2011
  613.2—dc23
                                  2011016579

Printed in Canada

10   9   8   7   6   5   4   3   2   1

Contents

KILLER COLAS

Introduction

Many years ago, I caught my children shaking cans of soda so that they would explode upon opening. I remember yelling at them for wasting the soft drinks. Knowing what I know now about the terrible toll that these beverages can take on your health, I think I should have showered my kids with gifts instead. These days, unfortunately, soda isn't the only drink that can ruin your health and the health of your children. The industry has branched out, offering numerous products that can get you hooked and lead to illness, including sports drinks, energy drinks, iced teas, and enhanced waters. Temptation is everywhere and comes in many different bottles and cans. *Killer Colas* is designed to help you resist temptation by providing you with the hard facts about soda and other sweetened beverages.

The book begins by explaining how important internal balance is to your health and how food items such as soda throw your body out of balance, leading to frailty and disease over time. It then provides a brief history of the soft drink industry, illustrating how soda became such a fixture in modern society, from its humble origins in pharmacies around the country to its transformation into one of the largest commercial enterprises in the world. Once you understand the big picture, you'll read about the dirty details of soft drinks and other sweetened beverages. Chapter 3 will tell you exactly what you are putting into your body when drinking these products, and Chapter 4 will describe the most common types of beverages in which these troublesome ingredients are found.

From there, it's time to learn about the many links between sweetened drinks and the numerous deadly diseases and health conditions that have been plaguing society in recent years. With connections to health problems such as asthma, allergies, heart disease, and even cancer, the goods sold by soda corporations may cost you far more than the change in your pocket. Sadly, even when you realize the dangers of these products, they can be much harder to quit than you'd think. In fact, soft drinks can result in addiction in much the same way that alcohol and some illegal street drugs do, as outlined in Chapter 6. In addition to this obstacle, the soft drink industry markets its drinks on a massive scale, making temptation very hard to avoid. Whether they are straightforward or a little sneaky, advertisements for sweetened beverages are virtually inescapable, as you will learn in Chapter 7. Thankfully, *Killer Colas* is here to help.

While soda consumption can be a habit that seems almost impossible to break, there are ways to get the monkey off your back, all of which you will read about in Chapter 8. Although the first step in this journey is yours alone to take, when your community provides education on the dangers of drinking soda and other sweetened beverages, and various levels of government support policies that promote a healthful diet, the chance of you taking two steps back is much less likely. If we all work together, the benefits that come from quitting soft drinks will be enjoyed not only by the individual but also by society at large. For your own sake and the sake of children everywhere, it is time to make a change.

The purpose of this book is to reveal the true cost of consuming soda and other sugary drinks. The following pages expose the scary facts about the many liquid refreshments marketed to the public by soft drink corporations. Whether you drink soft drinks on a regular basis or simply have one occasionally, *Killer Colas* will make you think twice before ever buying a soda or any type of sweetened beverage again.

1

Homeostasis and Body Chemistry

My journey towards wellness started over thirty years ago when I began to research my persistent ill health, which doctors couldn't seem to cure. I had contracted pneumonia many times and suffered from a whole list of allergy symptoms on a regular basis. I finally found the work of Melvin Page, Weston Price, Francis Pottenger, and Walter B. Cannon, from whom I learned variations of one simple truth: We cause a great majority of diseases ourselves through our diet, which has long since gone its separate way from the diet of our Stone Age ancestors.

The Paleolithic diet was made up of meat, vegetables, whole grains, nuts, mushrooms and other edible fungi, whole fruit, and water. Sugar as we now know it was never a part of the daily intake of food. This diet changed slowly with the advent of settled agriculture, but not enough to alter dramatically how often people got sick. And then, far too recently for evolution to allow humans to adapt to a high-sugar diet, we added sugar, which is now an overwhelmingly large part of our everyday eating habits. (See the inset "Sugary Stats" on page 6.)

YOUR BODY'S BALANCING ACT

Sugar, certainly in the amount that we eat today, can bring about problems in your body. This is because your system has to be in

5

Sugary Stats

Whether you call it pop, soda, soda pop, a soft drink, a carbonated drink, a cold drink, an energy drink, a sports drink, fruit juice, or a fruit drink, all of these beverages, if they are not sugar free, contain a lot of sugar and, usually, caffeine. If the drink is made with sugar and is in the amount of twelve ounces, which many soft drinks are, chances are you are getting about ten teaspoons, or forty grams, of sugar per serving. Fruit drinks, which have a maximum of only 5 percent of actual fruit, also have approximately ten teaspoons of added sugar. Even real fruit juice—including fresh apple, grape, and orange juice—contains about ten teaspoons of sugar in every twelve-ounce glass. Yes, it is naturally occurring sugar, but it upsets your body chemistry in the same way that added sugar does.

As of 2005, the average American drank a little over eight gallons of fruit juice, and close to thirty-six gallons of regular soft drinks (with sugar) per year. Let's see, that's a total of about forty-four gallons of drinks that at best should be called sugar water. That works out to approximately 379 twelve-ounce cans of soda and 87 twelve-ounce servings of fruit juice per person per year. As you can see, that is a little over twelve ounces of sugary drinks each day. Diet soda doesn't include sugar, but it does contain artificial sweeteners; and we drink 171

homeostasis in order to be healthy. *Homeostasis,* as coined by Dr. Cannon, is the process by which your body maintains a balance that allows it to work at peak efficiency. Glucose, blood urea nitrogen, uric acid, numerous minerals, and many other factors work in harmony with each other to keep you well. The sugar in your diet causes undesirable changes in your homeostatic system. Though it tries its best to adapt, the human body simply does not know how to handle the glut of sugar that we consume. This problem soon affects the minerals in your system, causing them to become unbalanced. Some of them become excessive and others become depleted. This imbalance can show up very well on a blood test after as little as two teaspoons of sugar are ingested.

cans of diet soda per person per year.[1] So, we drink more than 637 twelve-ounce cans of soda or glasses of juice every year. And please remember that this is an average; you probably drink more or you wouldn't be reading this book.

But you shouldn't just take my word that soft drinks will slowly kill you. In 2004, the American Association of Pediatrics (AAP) recommended that "pediatricians should work to eliminate sweetened drinks in schools." These doctors cited obesity, the lack of nutrients common to whole foods and milk (such as calcium), and dental erosion as the primary reasons behind this policy change. Some of the statistics used by the AAP in forming this policy statement, which all pediatricians are urged to follow, include the fact that each twelve-ounce can of soda ingested daily is associated with an 0.18 increase in a child's body mass index (BMI) number and a 60-percent increase in obesity risk. Particularly, these increases were thought to be caused by ingesting sugar energy in liquid form.

This is just the beginning of the scary stuff. Remember that there are over 3,000 different sugary drinks made just here in the United States. There are also fruit drinks, energy drinks, and sport drinks to consider, without even mentioning drinks ending in "ade," such as lemonade, or cocktail mixes. I will briefly discuss each major drink category in Chapter 4.

A BODY OUT OF WHACK

The fact is that all the minerals in your body are supposed to work in concert. The Mineral Wheel on page 8 shows the interconnected nature of your body's most important minerals. As displayed by the spokes in the wheel, each mineral promotes or inhibits the activity of another. In order for these processes to occur properly, your body must maintain a sufficient amount of each element. This delicate balance is thrown out of whack every time you eat sugar, which disrupts your overall homeostasis. When you are no longer in homeostasis, the progression of disease soon begins.

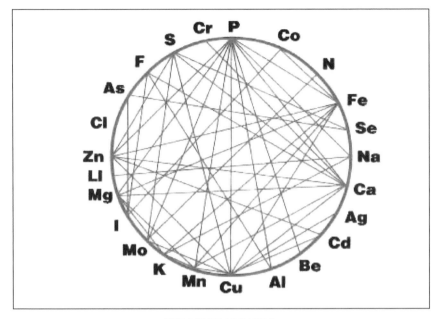

THE MINERAL WHEEL
Minerals work only when they are in proper relation to one another.

Calcium depletion is a prime example of a mineral imbalance caused by sugar. To explain, sugar makes your blood acidic. In reaction to this acidity, calcium is pulled from your bones in an effort to bring your body back to an alkaline state of homeostasis. This process soon leads to excessive calcium in your bloodstream. The calcium in your blood is then excreted in your urine, making your bones calcium-deficient and leading to osteoporosis.

EXHAUSTING YOUR IMMUNE SYSTEM

When you become deficient in minerals, your digestive enzymes cannot work as well. Unfortunately, when they cannot work as well, your food is not digested completely. This partially digested food results in unusable protein molecules and other particles, which get into your bloodstream where they do not belong. Your immune system sees the partially digested food as a foreign invader, like a bacteria or virus, and escorts the foreign invader out of the body. Unfortunately, your immune system was not meant to do this on a daily basis, and so it becomes exhausted. An immune system that is not working well opens the door to infectious and degenerative diseases.

CONCLUSION

Studies have linked sugar—including sucrose, fructose, and high fructose corn syrup—to diabetes, obesity, heart disease, stroke, and cancer. It doesn't matter whether it's Coke, Red Bull, Gatorade, or Hi-C. The glut of liquid sugar consumed without the fiber of whole fruit hits the bloodstream running, causing a suppressed immune system and eventually disease, the effects of which will be discussed in Chapter 5. While the primary reason to avoid sweetened drinks in our diet is sugar, sometimes sugar is taken out of these drinks and substituted with a non-caloric sweetener. Soft drink manufacturers have made billions from the sale of diet drinks that may have fewer calories than the regular versions but are no better for you, as also revealed in Chapter 5.

But before you learn about all of the potentially harmful ingredients in these deadly drinks, it is important to first take a brief history lesson and find out exactly how soda became the massive industry it is today.

2

How Did We Get Here?

When I wrote *Lick the Sugar Habit* in 1986, the average American was consuming about 142 pounds of sugar a year. Soda and other sugary drinks represented half or more of that statistic, depending on the segment of the population under discussion. With obesity rates now skyrocketing, what we really want to know is this: When did major soda makers such as Coca-Cola and Pepsi first learn that their products were generally harmful, and have they been covering up these facts? Sadly, the answers are most likely buried deep in corporate memos. I suppose Big Soda learned from Big Tobacco not to leave such damaging memos in the hands of possibly disgruntled employees who may later turn whistleblowers.

The only other way to discover what these documents might say about the health consequences of soda (which include increased obesity, diabetes, cancer, heart disease, and the many other diseases touched on in Chapter 5) would be to sue someone. For a trial to proceed, however, plaintiffs must show initial grounds for a lawsuit. Big Tobacco was finally brought to court after years of clear government-funded research that directly linked smoking to cancer. Only after the public's views were changed by repeated instruction in the media did the whistleblowers appear with memos that told the tale of nicotine enhancement, massive ad campaigns conducted by cynical executives, and political contributions that served to delay the prosecution of tobacco companies for decades.

So far, the public hasn't fully accepted the fact that soda is bad for you, in part because the major soda companies fund their own research and may have influenced the results of the studies. There has been no big groundswell against soda (or any other sugary drink, for that matter) to justify a lawsuit that would release internal documents. Of course, it could be that Big Soda is a slightly different industry than Big Tobacco—that it is ignorant rather than callously peddling an addiction. But, in my experience, companies that become billion-dollar enterprises within the space of approximately 120 years aren't generally in the dark about their core product.

On the contrary, they usually guard information about their products quite closely. For example, Coca-Cola's original recipe is treated like freshly issued nuclear codes. Only two executives may know the secret recipe at one time, and so are forbidden to fly together in the same aircraft for fear that the knowledge might be lost in a crash. There is certainly a lot of effort involved in making billions off your soft drink habit, don't you think?

Nevertheless, right now, we can only guess what Big Soda knows and when it first came to know it. There is, however, always the tantalizing possibility that we will one day learn that Big Soda is not our friend, no matter how much money it provides to worthy charities and schools. But before we imagine the future, it is time for a little history lesson.

THE BIRTH OF AN INDUSTRY

So how did we get here? Did it begin in 1798, with the first recorded usage of soda water; or in 1819, with the first patent for the soda fountain? I suppose, for most people, a convenient starting place would be 1886, when Atlanta pharmacist John Pemberton invented Coca-Cola. (See the inset "A Soda Timeline" on page 14.) Pemberton, however, didn't invent the drink as we know it today.

His health failed within a year of inventing a syrup that contained sugar, kola nut extract (a caffeine source), and coca leaf extract (cocaine), which was actually intended as a health concoction. (Please take a moment to appreciate the irony that the inventor of this "health syrup" had to sell his business due to illness.) Coca-Cola's early years then continued under Willis Venable, another pharmacist, who added the carbonated water.

Scientists had discovered that carbon dioxide was behind the bubbles in natural mineral water. Shortly after that, it seemed like a good idea not only to bathe in mineral water but also to drink it. Because the water seemed to have curative powers, the first sodas appeared in drug store soda fountains. To give the beverage an appealing flavor, pharmacists decided to add herbs to the soda water, including birch bark, dandelion, sarsaparilla, and fruit extracts. After a while, the public liked to drink the bubbly water so much that its actual mineral content became much less important. The soda fountain soon took its place in popular culture. Before long, customers wanted to take their favorite fizzy drink home, and so the soft drink bottling industry was born.

Venable's next contribution to the story of Coca-Cola was the realization that he couldn't sell his product properly. He sold the business to Asa Chandler, who was responsible for the birth of the soft drink corporation as we know it. His business model—which kept the syrup in-house, franchised the bottling, and relentlessly advertised the product—created huge profits and exponential growth. By 1904, due to an advertising budget that equaled 25 percent of the company's total income, Coca-Cola was the most recognized brand in America.

THE COLA WARS

Coca-Cola's trademarks and symbols remain some of the most recognizable images in the world, alongside Jesus, Elvis Presley, and Superman. Coca-Cola's marketing and promotional budgets have ballooned well past $3 billion a year. Although, it must be said, the company doesn't direct 25 percent of its earnings

A Soda Timeline

1767. English theologian, natural philosopher, and political theorist Joseph Priestley invents carbonated water.

1770. Swedish chemist Torbern Bergman discovers a way to make carbonated water from chalk.

1798. Sodium salts, which are added to create carbonated mineral water, cause the term "soda water" to be coined.

1810. The process of mass-producing artificial mineral water receives a United States patent.

1819. Pennsylvania native Samuel Fahnestock invents the soda fountain.

1835. Bottled soda water begins to be sold in the United States.

1851. Dr. Thomas Cantrell invents ginger ale in Ireland.

1871. The first United States trademark registration is given to Lemon's Superior Sparkling Ginger Ale.

1874. Robert M. Green invents the ice cream soda in Philadelphia.

1876. Root beer begins to be mass produced for public consumption.

1881. The first cola-flavored soda appears on the market.

1885. Pharmacist Charles Alderton creates Dr Pepper in Waco, Texas.

1886. Pharmacist John S. Pemberton invents Coca-Cola in Atlanta, Georgia. It is conceived as a headache remedy.

1892. Inventor William Painter invents the bottle cap, the first bottle stopper to preserve the carbonation of soda water.

1895. Coca-Cola debuts its first print ad, featuring actress Hilda Clark as its first spokesperson.

1899. A glass-blowing machine is patented and used in the production of glass bottles. Within a few years, glass bottle production increases from 1,500 bottles a day to 57,000 bottles a day.

1903. Pepsi-Cola, created as a cure for dyspepsia (heartburn and stomach ache), is trademarked.

1905. Still marketed as a tonic, Coca-Cola removes extracts of cocaine from their drink.

1913. Delivery vehicles progress from horse-drawn carriages to gas-powered trucks.

1914–1918. World War I slows down production of soft drinks due to sugar rationing.

1916. White Castle becomes the first fast-food chain, setting in motion the explosion of fast-food restaurants of the 1940s and 1950s. These restaurants became huge money makers for the soft drink industry.

1920. Prohibition begins, giving soft drinks a big push. It is around this time that vending machines begin dispensing soda into cups.

1923. Six-pack cardboard cartons called "Hom-Paks" are introduced to carry soft drinks home.

1929. Charles Leiper Grigg creates a lemon-lime soft drink called Bib-Label Lithiated Lemon-Lime Soda in St. Louis. It is later renamed 7 Up.

1933. Prohibition ends and soft drinks lose their popularity to hard drinks. It is also the beginning of mixed drinks (soft drinks mixed with alcohol).

1939. Pepsi-Cola begins selling its beverage in twelve-ounce bottles, compared to the six-ounce and eight-ounce bottles preferred by the competition.

1940–1945. During World War II, soft drinks are given to soldiers at no cost. (What a great way to get lots of servicemen hooked.)

1952. The first diet soft drink, a ginger ale called No-Cal, is sold by Kirsch Beverages.

1963. Diet cola Slenderella is packaged using the first aluminum soda can.

1965. Vending machines begin to offer soft drinks in aluminum cans, which soon dominate the market.

1970. Soft drinks are sold in plastic bottles for the first time.

1977. The United States significantly increases the cost of imported sugar. Seeking a cheaper sweetener for their products, soda producers begin using high-fructose corn syrup (HFCS).

1979. Mello Yello soft drink is introduced in certain areas of the country by the Coca-Cola Company as competition against Mountain Dew. The company plans on expanding its availability throughout the United States.

2003. California becomes the first state to ban the sale of soda in elementary, middle, and junior high schools.

2006. Several major soft drink companies in the United States agree to limit the sale of soda in public schools.

2009. The New York City Department of Health launches a massive advertising campaign called "Pouring on the Pounds," which warns about the dangers of soda and other sugary drinks.

towards advertising anymore, spending closer to 10 percent these days. Perhaps it doesn't have to spend quite so much because its product is so firmly entrenched in American society. Marketing, however, will always be at the forefront of Coca-Cola's business strategy, especially when its biggest rival is nipping at its heels.

Pepsi was the second major entry into the cola and soda market, starting in 1898. Caleb Bradham's company limped along, declaring bankruptcy twice before 1931. Pepsi recovered and expanded abroad just like Coke, but spent many years in its competitor's shadow. World War II highlighted the disparity between the two companies, as Coke got the contract to supply drinks to the United States military, which came with exemptions from the sugar rationing imposed by the government in 1942. Pepsi had to make do without the contract, limited to the domestic market, until the war ended.

By this time, the practice of basically giving away Coca-Cola to soldiers during the war had created a customer base that took the Pepsi corporation decades to crack. Pepsi began to close the gap in market share during the 1960s by acquiring non-cola brands like Mountain Dew, Mug Root Beer, and many others that are now proudly listed on its website. Pepsi then expanded into fast-food restaurants, creating captive venues for its drink at Taco Bell, Kentucky Fried Chicken, and Pizza Hut, until these fast-food chains were spun off into another company in 1997. Pepsi also purchased and still holds the Frito-Lay company, the premier snack food producer in America. Coke may have dominated soda throughout the 1970s, but Pepsi's diversification kept it in the game as it waited for its big moment. That big moment was the Pepsi Challenge.

During the 1980s, the Pepsi Challenge, a possibly rigged taste-test campaign, broke down the old patterns of the long-standing Coke-Pepsi grudge match. Suddenly, Coke was on the defensive for having a slightly less sweet cola. It appeared as though Pepsi had made Coke blink. Coke changed its formula, and comedian Bill Cosby, the Coca-Cola spokesman at the time, touted the new

Coke with the same aplomb as he did the old Coke. The change, however, was a disaster. About five years later, Coke declared a return to the old formula, now called Classic Coke. Market research had shown that the people who wanted a Coke didn't want the drink to mimic Pepsi so closely. Sales increased, and Bill Cosby continued to tell us to "have a Coke and a smile."

CONCLUSION

So who won the Coke-Pepsi rumble? The truth is that it continues unabated. And I'm sure there is more to be discovered about how the two largest dinosaurs on the field of battle do business. If the relevant corporate documents are ever released, perhaps all the answers to our questions will finally be revealed. Right now, all I can tell you for certain is that many of these drinks are addictive and have serious health consequences. And yet, they are readily available. Even the size of soda containers has grown considerably. The bottom line is this: Any company that sells an addictive substance and increases the availability of that substance can never be your friend.

3

The Ingredients

Do you know what is in your favorite drink? The answer is not rocket science, but it does help to have a primer so you can decode the ingredient labels of soft drinks and other sugary beverages. Basically, the main ingredients in soft drinks are carbonated water, sweetener, phosphoric acid, artificial and natural flavorings, caffeine, and preservatives. But you can simplify that list further to read carbonated water, sweetener, and chemicals. Other sweetened beverages, such as sports drinks and energy drinks, usually contain similar ingredients, along with additives that include herbs, vitamins, and minerals, which are supposed to make these drinks seem healthful. The following chapter explains these commonly used ingredients in greater detail, from natural and artificial sweeteners to herbs and chemical additives. Once you have learned more about these substances, the choice to continue drinking the products that contain them is yours.

COMMON SWEETENERS

There are many ways to make a beverage sweet. Some of them are natural, some of them are artificial, but all of them have an effect on your body. The following examples are some of the most common sweeteners used in the beverage industry.

Table Sugar (Sucrose)

Derived from sugar beets or cane, table sugar, also known as sucrose, was the first major sugar to be used as a sweetener in whole and processed foods. It is made up of two simple sugars, also known as *monosaccharides,* called glucose and fructose. These simple sugars occur in equal proportion and are chemically bound together in sucrose. This slows their absorption in your body, allowing your system to metabolize them a little bit at a time. Glucose is ultimately metabolized throughout your body with the help of insulin, while fructose is processed only by your liver.

High-Fructose Corn Syrup (HFCS)

Starting in the 1970s, enterprising drink manufacturers replaced sucrose with high-fructose corn syrup (HFCS), as it was cheaper to grow corn, a local grain, than to import sugar cane, which grows in tropical and subtropical climates. But is there really a difference between high-fructose corn syrup and table sugar when it comes to your body? Research has shown that HFCS does, in fact, affect your body differently than regular sugar, in both the short-term and the long-term.

In one study, rats who consumed high-fructose corn syrup along with their regular food gained significantly more weight than those that had their normal diets supplemented with table sugar, even though the caloric intake was the same in both groups.[1] In addition, the long-term consumption of high-fructose corn syrup led to abnormal increases in body fat, especially around the abdomen. Finally, HFCS was also associated with a rise in triglycerides, which are a type of fat found in your blood. According to Princeton University Professor Bart Hoebel, while some people claim that high-fructose corn syrup affects weight gain in the same way as any other sweetener, this study suggests a different conclusion. High-fructose corn syrup is associated with obesity more frequently than table sugar or even a high-fat diet. This may have something to do with the chemical composition of HFCS.

While table sugar is consists of 50 percent glucose and 50 percent fructose, high-fructose corn syrup is typically made up of 42 percent glucose and 55 percent fructose, with larger sugar molecules called *higher saccharides* accounting for the remaining 3 percent. In addition, the fructose and glucose molecules in HFCS are not bound together as they are in sucrose, which causes them to be metabolized rapidly, increasing the burden on your system. In particular, the elevated level and form of fructose contained in high-fructose corn syrup is thought to promote health problems more easily than the fructose found in table sugar.

Although all the differences between HFCS and table sugar are not yet fully understood, scientists believe that excess fructose is metabolized to produce fat, while excess glucose is processed for energy or stored as a carbohydrate called *glycogen.* Unfortunately, since the 1970s, when research began to show a relationship between sugar and disease, we have not only increased the amount of sugar we eat but also added more fructose to our diet. Not long after this research was published, however, Snapple, a sugary fruit drink made by Pepsi, switched its sweetener from high-fructose corn syrup back to table sugar. I think this change could very well be the tip of the iceberg, and that many more beverage companies will go back to using sucrose in their products.

Maltodextrin

Similar in appearance to table sugar, maltodextrin is slightly less sweet than sucrose and has fewer calories, which makes it ideal for sports drinks. It can also add a unique smooth texture to a beverage. Although it can also be made from rice or potatoes, maltodextrin is primarily made from corn. Unfortunately, maltodextrin spikes insulin and glucose levels more than sugar and high-fructose corn syrup. It throws your body out of homeostasis rapidly, making your system work hard to get back in balance. Stay away from this product.

Crystalline Fructose

Like HFCS, crystalline fructose is derived from corn, though it is processed in a way that makes it almost entirely fructose. While HFCS generally contains 55 percent fructose, crystalline fructose is made up of at least 98 percent pure fructose. So, basically everything that is wrong with high-fructose corn syrup simply gets heightened at this level of purity. Crystalline fructose is not a good thing to put into your body. This fact may cause beverage manufacturers to switch back to high-fructose corn syrup, or perhaps even sucrose, as a sweetener for their drinks.

Honey

Honey is the sweet, thick liquid that bees produce from plant nectar. Most honey is approximately 20 percent water, 40 percent fructose, 30 percent glucose, and 1 percent sucrose. The small remainder is a combination of other sugars and minute traces of naturally present acids, vitamins, minerals, and enzymes. Honey from different locations can vary in composition and flavor, depending on the type of flowering plant from which the bees take the nectar. (Bees can get their nectar from over 300 plants.) Three of the most common sources of nectar are clover, orange blossom, and sage.

Maple Syrup

Maple syrup is created by boiling the sap of sugar maple, red maple, or black maple trees, which causes some of the water content to evaporate, thus concentrating the sugar. Maple sugar generally contains about 33 percent water and 60 percent sucrose. The remainder is a mixture of small amounts of glucose and fructose, minute traces of naturally present acids and minerals, as well as some B vitamins.

SUGAR SUBSTITUTES

Whether they are low calorie or calorie free, natural or artificial, sugar substitutes are additives that attempt to match the taste of sugar-based sweeteners in a food or drink. Many of the following sweeteners are controversial, with arguments both for and against their use. Before approving sweeteners such as aspartame, acesulfame potassium, saccharin, sucralose, and neotame, the FDA reviewed more than 100 safety studies to determine their effect on human health. Although some research showed negative consequences associated with these products, there were enough positive results for the FDA to clear the sweeteners for general use. A number of experts, however, feel that many of the positive results came from questionable tests.

Side effects of some of these artificial sweeteners have been reported to include an increase in the number of migraine headaches experienced by migraine sufferers[2] as well as the chronic pain of fibromyalgia.[3] As of yet, however, the FDA has found no clear association between these substances and cancer risk in humans or any other threat to human health.[4] Despite these claims, there are many consumer groups and professionals in the field of health and nutrition who have devoted themselves to exposing the health problems caused by artificial sweeteners. Much of this information, although not generally peer-reviewed, is learned firsthand by practitioners through their experiences with patients. (For more information on the groups that are dedicated to exposing the truth about artificial sweetners, see the Resources on page 103.)

As far as I am concerned, artificial sweeteners are not whole foods. The body has a harder time dealing with some of the substances in these sweeteners, and the whole system has to work harder to either eliminate them or turn them into a substance that the body can use. I see no reason to put them in our bodies.

Whatever your thoughts are on the matter, it has been proven that certain people are more prone to the potential negative effects of artificial sweeteners than others. These people include diabetics, children, women of childbearing age, pregnant and breastfeeding women, individuals with low seizure thresholds, and those who suffer from migraines.

What follows next are some of the most common sugar substitutes. Brief explanations of these products along with their most popular brand names are provided.

Acesulfame Potassium, Acesulfame K, Ace K (Sweet One, Sunett)

Acesulfame is made from a process involving acetoacetic acid (a weak acid) and potassium. It is usually used in combination with aspartame or sucralose, both of which help decrease its bitter aftertaste to create a taste that is close to actual sugar. Although the FDA feels otherwise, some say that this product could be carcinogenic and warrants better research.

Aspartame (NutraSweet, Equal)

Aspartame consists of methanol and the amino acids aspartic acid and phenylalanine. These components are not toxic to your system, but when they break down during the process of manufacturing and transportation, from sitting on the shelf in a store or your home, or through the metabolic process in your body, they can turn into harmful substances.

Methanol, for instance, can spontaneously break down into formaldehyde, also a toxin, which can accumulate in your cells and cause health problems. Phenylalinine, when stored at warm temperatures or for an extended period of time, turns into diketopiperazine, a known carcinogen. And for those who have phenylketonuria (PKU), an inherited disease in which the body is unable to properly metabolize phenylalanine, this chemical is an obvious health hazard.

Although numerous studies have confirmed the safety of this product, the source of the research must be questioned. According to a survey of 166 studies on aspartame, Dr. Robert Walton found that 74 had been funded by the aspartame industry, all of which reported this sweetener as safe. Of the 92 remaining studies, nearly all suggested major health concerns with the product.[5]

Neotame

While neotame is chemically similar to aspartame, its composition is different enough so that it is not a source of phenylalanine. It is metabolized rapidly and seems to leave no trace in the body. Although it has been shown to be safe for human consumption in a large number of studies, its relationship to aspartame still arouses suspicion in critics who worry about its rising popularity as an additive.

Saccharin (Sweet'N Low)

Originally used as an antiseptic and a food preservative, saccharin began its use as a food sweetener during the sugar shortages of World War I and World War II. It is not metabolized by the body and has no effect on blood sugar levels. Although its safety has come under scrutiny in the past, the National Toxicology Program (NTP) removed saccharin from the list of potential carcinogens in 1997. There are still, however, many researchers and consumer organizations that feel not enough long-term research has been done on this artificial sweetener.

Sucralose (Splenda)

The name sucralose is misleading. The suffix "ose" is used to name natural sweeteners such as fructose, glucose, and sucrose, not artificial additives. And because sucralose sounds very close to sucrose (table sugar), the name can be confusing.

Sugar is used in the production of sucralose, but the two are very different substances. The manufacturing process of sucralose chemically substitutes chlorine atoms in place of hydrogen-oxygen atom groups on the sugar molecule. Once it reaches the gut, the body does not recognize it as food, therefore it has no calories. Although, the sucralose sold in packets under the brand name Splenda is actually mixed with a bulking ingredient such as dextrose or maltodextrin, which makes it appear and taste more like table sugar but also adds a few calories.

Check Those Labels!

"No sugar" or "sugar free," "naturally sweetened," "all natural," "no added sugar." These are common terms found on many commercial foods and beverages. But what do they actually mean?

If the label says:	It means:
No sugar / Sugar free	The product does not contain any natural sweeteners such as sucrose (table sugar), high-fructose corn syrup, honey, or maple syrup. It may contain sugar alcohols or artificial sweeteners.
No added sugar	No extra natural sweeteners were added during processing. Before processing, however, the original source of the product may have contained sugar, such as fructose in fruit juice. Also, sugar alcohols or artificial sweeteners may have been added.
Naturally sweetened / All natural	The product does not contain any artificial ingredients. It may contain natural sweeteners, such as sucrose (table sugar), high-fructose corn syrup, honey, or maple syrup. It may also contain sugar alcohols.

Steviol Glycosides (Stevia, Sweet Leaf, Honey Leaf, Only Sweet, PureVia)

A natural sugar substitute extracted from the stevia leaf, steviol glycosides are becoming more and more popular since the FDA allowed these extracts to be categorized as sweeteners in 2008. Although stevia extracts can be up to 300 times as sweet as regular sugar, they have virtually no effect on blood sugar. Additionally, no major side effects, allergies, or physical or mental harm have been reported in medical journals from their use. Steviol glycosides are safe for use by diabetics, sufferers of phenylketonuria, and individuals who are trying to lose weight.[6]

Although stevia seems to have no downside, the reality is that it tastes sweet (like all sugar substitutes). And if you are addicted to sugar, this sweetness will keep your craving for sugar alive. It will have you coming back for more sweet foods and drinks, sometimes in any form. I do not believe it is ever a good idea to use steviol glycosides or any other form of sweetener. Essentially, you make the task of quitting sugar harder by using other sweeteners. They simply prolong your addiction instead of end it.

Sugar Alcohols

Common sugar alcohols include sorbitol, xylitol, malitol, erythritol, and mannitol. Those that are naturally occurring are extracted from the fiber of a number of fruits and vegetables. This extraction process, however, is not commercially viable, so sugar alcohols are now created by adding hydrogen to simple sugars such as glucose, fructose, and maltose. Their chemical structure is part sugar, part alcohol, though technically they are neither a sugar nor an alcohol. These sweeteners have about half the calories of table sugar and do not trigger an insulin reaction. They are not, however, completely digested by the small intestine, which is their major drawback. As a result, they can ferment in the intestine and cause diarrhea, irritable bowel syndrome, bloating, stomach rumbling, and flatulence in some people.

OTHER ADDITIVES

In addition to sweeteners, the makers of soft drinks and other sugary beverages use numerous other additives in the creation of their products. Whether they are added to carbonate a drink, preserve it, or manipulate its flavor and color, these additives may not just enhance the look and taste of a beverage, they may also affect your health.

Phosphoric Acid

After sweeteners, phosphoric acid may have the biggest impact on your health. Soft drink manufacturers add this chemical to soda to give it a tangy flavor and maintain its carbonation until popping the top releases the gas. Basic high school science should tell you that phosphoric acid introduces phosphorus to the bloodstream. Remember the importance of mineral balance that I mentioned in Chapter 1? Good, you're paying attention.

Sugar consumption usually creates a drop in phosphorus and a rise in calcium, disturbing their proper ratio. The appearance of more calcium and less phosphorus in the body results in lots of calcium sitting around doing nothing. This excess calcium can turn into plaque that negatively affects the teeth, eyes, and blood vessels. It would seem logical to add phosphorus to counteract these normal conditions of sugar consumption. But even if powering down a Coke to counteract the chocolate cake you ate could work, you must remember that you're getting phosphorus along with sugar, caffeine, and other chemicals, which all work in separate ways to suppress your immune system. In addition, similar health effects come from having too much phosphorus in the bloodstream.

Phosphoric acid is one nasty chemical. It raises phosphorus in the blood stream so much that it changes the pH of the body, making it highly acidic, which is another stress upon the system. If you think battery acid splashed on skin is a serious injury, so too is excess phosphoric acid on your internal structures. Most immune systems will simply go on strike in such a highly acidic environment. Sodium, potassium, magnesium, and calcium are all called upon to put the body back in a slightly alkaline state, also known as homeostasis. As a result, all minerals may become depleted by the effect of phosphoric acid in soda. These mineral depletions can lead to diseases that include colitis, arthritis, kidney stones, and arterial plaque, as well as digestive problems, as you will see in Chapter 5. Many non-alcoholic beverages contain phosphoric acid, and fruit juices contain natural acids, which may have similar effects.

Caffeine

Caffeine is a stimulant with mild addictive properties. Whether it comes from the natural concentrations found in kola nuts and coffee beans, or is purposely added for flavor, caffeine will always leave you wanting more. Once you're hooked, it is hard to say no. Overuse of caffeine can lead to heart palpitations, anxiety, and insomnia, to name but a few possible side effects. To learn the

Caffeine Content

The list below details the caffeine content of some of the most popular name-brand drinks on the market, as well as coffee and tea. Products are listed from those containing the least amount of caffeine to the most.

Trade Name	Quantity	Caffeine
Slim-Fast Chocolate Flavors	12 fluid ounces	20 mg
A & W Cream Soda	12 fluid ounces	29 mg
Snapple Flavored Teas	12 fluid ounces	31.5 mg
Coca-Cola Classic	12 fluid ounces	34 mg
Diet Pepsi	12 fluid ounces	36 mg
Pepsi-Cola	12 fluid ounces	37.5 mg
Dr Pepper	12 fluid ounces	41 mg
Diet Dr Pepper	12 fluid ounces	41 mg
RC Cola	12 fluid ounces	43 mg
Diet Coke	12 fluid ounces	45.6 mg
Tab	12 fluid ounces	46.8 mg
Mountain Dew	12 fluid ounces	55 mg
Diet Mountain Dew	12 fluid ounces	55 mg
Pepsi One	12 fluid ounces	55.5 mg
Jolt	12 fluid ounces	71.2 mg
Full Throttle Fury	8 fluid ounces	72 mg
Hype Energy Drink	8 fluid ounces	77 mg
Red Bull	8.2 fluid ounces	80 mg
Spike Shooter	8.4 fluid ounces	300 mg

amount of caffeine contained in some of the most popular drinks on the market, see the inset "Caffeine Content" on page 29.

Guarana

Found in the Amazon rain forest, guarana is a plant whose seeds contain roughly double the amount of caffeine found in coffee beans. It forms the basis of many South American sodas and is beginning to be used in energy drinks and teas in North America. The risks of this specific ingredient are not known, as it has not been evaluated by the FDA for safety, effectiveness, or purity. The information on guarana's side effects comes from what is known about caffeine, but the substance itself has not yet been adequately studied.

Yerba Maté

Like guarana, yerba maté is a plant native to South America that contains caffeine. Although many praise it as healthful, others point to evidence that it may actually be carcinogenic. Because of its caffeine content, its side effects can include heartbeat irregularities, trouble sleeping, and nervousness. Yerba maté, therefore, should be avoided by people taking drugs that act as stimulants, including asthma medications and diet pills such as ephedrine.

Carbon Dioxide

Carbonated water—also known as soda, soda water, sparkling water, fizzy water, and seltzer—is plain water (most likely filtered from a municipal source) in which carbon dioxide gas has been dissolved. The process of carbonation is the main component of soft drinks, and the release of this gas is responsible for the popping sound you hear when you open a soft drink container.

In addition to the bubbles in the water, however, carbonation results in the formation of carbonic acid. Along with the phosphoric acid of soda water, carbonic acid increases the acidity of a drink, which helps prevent the growth of mold, yeast, and lactic acid bacteria. Measured on the pH scale—on which 0 signifies a completely acidic solution, 7 signifies a neutral solution, and 14 signifies a completely alkaline solution—the pH level of most soft drinks falls between the acidic range of 3 and 4. Unfortunately, this high acidity also depletes the calcium in your bones, which your body releases to bring itself back into acid-alkaline balance.

Caramel Coloring

Although it may sound harmless, the caramel coloring used to give colas such as Coke and Pepsi a more palatable appearance actually deserves a closer look. Created by the reaction of sugar with both ammonium and sulfite compounds, this particular type of caramel coloring is technically called Caramel IV, being the fourth of four kinds to be federally regulated. The process of manufacturing Caramel IV results in by-products such as 2-methylimidazole and 4-methylimidazole, both of which have demonstrated an association with lung, liver, and thyroid tumors in laboratory rats and mice.[7] Furthermore, the state of California has added 4-methylimidazole on its list of known carcinogens.

Research done at the University of California at Davis has shown that certain colas contain levels of 4-methylimidazole that far exceed the accepted limit. Unless this method of producing caramel coloring is banned, companies such as Coca-Cola and Pepsi should be forced to include warning labels on their colas.[8] At this point, it really seems like a no-brainer to find another coloring source.

Citric Acid

Naturally occurring in citrus fruits and berries, citric acid is added to fruit-flavored soft drinks to give them a tangy flavor. It also acts as a preservative.

Sodium Citrate

Sodium citrate is often included alongside citric acid to regulate the acidity of a soda. It also keeps any fats or fat-soluble compounds emulsified in the liquid. Because it is both salty and tart, it is also called "sour salt."

Ascorbic Acid

A form of vitamin C, ascorbic acid not only restores some of the nutritional value lost during the processing of a beverage but also acts as an antioxidant that helps improve the color and taste of a drink. It is most often used in soft drinks made with fruit juices. Ascorbic acid may, however, cause harm when it is added to a drink that contains the preservative sodium benzoate. The combination, when subjected to heat and light, results in the production of a carcinogen known as *benzene*. (For additional information, see "Sodium Benzoate" below.)

Flavoring

Of course, one of the most important aspects of soft drinks is flavoring. Most soda manufacturers mix a number of individual flavors together to create distinctive tastes for their drinks. In addition to artificial flavors, soft drinks use natural flavors that come from spices, herbs, and oils. Fruit-flavored soft drinks, such as orange and lemon-lime, often contain natural fruit extracts. Other beverages such as root beer and ginger ale contain flavoring made from plant roots.

Sodium Benzoate

Sodium benzoate is a preservative used by soft drink manufacturers to prevent the growth of organisms such as mold and bacteria in their products. As mentioned in the section on ascorbic acid, sodium benzoate is the source of incredible controversy. This controversy stems from the fact that the combination of ascorbic acid and sodium benzoate produces the carcinogenic compound known as benzene when subjected to high temperatures. Although the FDA has put a limit on the amount of benzoate that can be used in a product, many of the sodas on grocery shelves have been found to contain more than the designated amount. Interestingly, independent laboratory tests have found benzene in numerous brand-name soft drinks at levels above the federal limit.

I am not sure you should have any benzoate or benzene in your body at all. Although data from medical research suggests that benzoate poses no threat to human health in the amount found in a soft drink, I am not convinced. What if you drink three or four soft drinks? Then what?

Ginkgo Biloba

Traditionally used in Asian medicine and cooking, ginkgo biloba is a plant whose extract is commonly added to energy drinks. It is said to offer many benefits, such as enhanced memory and concentration, but is not without possible side effects. These side effects include nausea, dizziness, heart palpitations, and increased risk of bleeding. Therefore, ginkgo should not be taken by people on blood-thinning medication or women who are pregnant without the approval of a doctor.

Ginseng

Like ginkgo biloba, ginseng is an herb that has been used for its medicinal properties for many years throughout Asia. And like ginkgo biloba, little medical research has been done on ginseng. While it reportedly boosts brain power and reduces mental fatigue, it has also been associated with such side effects as headaches, nausea, and an inability to sleep.

Bisphenol A (BPA)

Although it is not technically an additive, Bisphenol A (BPA) is a chemical that may be found in soft drinks, sports drinks, energy drinks, and any beverage that comes in plastic packaging. It is used in the production of polycarbonate plastics as well as epoxy resins. Most commonly found in beverage bottles, baby bottles, and the lining of aluminum cans, BPA is known to leach out of these containers, particularly when they are in contact with high-temperature or acidic liquids. When bisphenol A accumulates in the body, it can disrupt normal hormone function, resulting in health problems. Children are particularly sensitive to this chemical, which has been associated with numerous negative effects on childhood development. Although many manufacturers are switching to BPA-free packaging, it is still difficult to avoid this chemical completely.

CONCLUSION

Now that you have a better idea of the ingredients found in soft drinks and other sugary beverages, are you sure you still want to drink them? The hard truth is that the ingredients mentioned above are simply the most common ones. There are over 3,000 drinks manufactured in the United States alone—and they include ingredients too numerous to mention in this chapter. In addition to the dangers of both natural and artificial sweeteners, other additives may also result in health problems over time. Whether they come from plants or are created in a lab, these substances often lack proper long-term research into their possible side effects. Simply because it appears in a drink and is featured on the label doesn't mean an ingredient is completely safe.

The following chapter discusses the many different types of sugary drinks on the market and provides a detailed example of each, including a list of ingredients that you will now recognize. I believe that the more you understand these drinks, the less willing you will be to subject your body to them.

4

Soft Drinks and Other Sweetened Beverages

Pop quiz. Which of the following drinks is the worst for your health: sugar-sweetened soft drinks, diet soda, sports drinks, energy drinks, iced teas, fruit drinks, fruit juices, or meal replacements? This is where I admit that this is a trick question, because each of these liquid refreshments can affect healthy body chemistry, creating conditions that lead to disease.

In this chapter, I will present a short discussion of each beverage category and include a sample product along with its ingredients and nutrition facts. Remember, there are over 3,000 different non-alcoholic drinks in the United States alone, so what I have given is really just a sampling. If you do not find your drink of choice on the following pages, don't worry. Simply read its product label to find what it contains, and then look up the ingredients in Chapter 3 to discover exactly what you are putting in your body. At that point, you can decide whether or not you really want to drink it.

SOFT DRINKS

A soft drink is made with flavored carbonated water that has been sweetened, usually with either sugar or high-fructose corn syrup. Diet soda differs from regular soda only in its lack of sugar and high-fructose corn syrup, which are generally replaced with some form of low-calorie or non-calorie artificial sweetener. Although there seems to be new brands on the market all the time, the most common examples include aspartame (NutraSweet), saccharin (Sweet & Low), sucralose (Splenda), acesulfame K (Sunett), and stevia (Truvia).

As one of the most recognized soft drink brands in the world, Coca-Cola is the perfect example of a regular soda, while Diet Pepsi, a rival drink, can easily illustrate the nutritional values of the average diet soda.

COCA-COLA

INGREDIENTS

Carbonated water, high-fructose corn syrup, caramel color, phosphoric acid, natural flavors, and caffeine.

NUTRITION FACTS (20 FLUID OUNCES)

Calories: 240	Sodium: 75 milligrams
Carbohydrates: 65 grams	Protein: 0
Sugar: 65 grams	Caffeine: 57 milligrams
Total Fat: 0	

DIET PEPSI

INGREDIENTS

Carbonated water, caramel color, aspartame, phosphoric acid, potassium benzoate, caffeine, citric acid, natural flavor, and phenylketonurics (contains phenylalanine).

NUTRITION FACTS (20 FLUID OUNCES)

Calories: 0	Sodium: 60 milligrams
Carbohydrates: 0	Protein: 0
Sugar: 0	Caffeine: 59 milligrams
Total Fat: 0	

SPORT DRINKS

Like energy drinks and enhanced water, a sports drink can be considered a functional beverage, as it is designed for a specific purpose aside from just quenching your thirst. Sports drinks are for athletes, who, in addition to needing water for hydration, require various salts, minerals, and vitamins, which leach from the body during heavy perspiration. Sodium and potassium salts, called *electrolytes* because of their importance in nerve conduction, are often present in large quantities in these beverages. Sugar or high-fructose corn syrup is also added to turn the salty water into a sweet fruit-flavored drink. As you will see, though they may have fruit-inspired names, these products generally do not contain any real fruit juice.

When you think of sports drinks, the Gatorade brand most likely comes to mind. The following example is one of Gatorade's most popular flavors.

GATORADE ORIGINAL LEMON-LIME

INGREDIENTS

Water, sucrose syrup, glucose-fructose syrup, citric acid, natural lemon and lime flavors with other natural flavors, salt, sodium citrate, monopotassium phosphate, ester gum, yellow 5.

NUTRITION FACTS (32 FLUID OUNCES)

Calories: 200

Carbohydrates: 56 grams

Sugar: 56 grams

Total Fat: 0

Sodium: 440 milligrams

Potassium: 120 milligrams

Protein: 0

ENERGY DRINKS

Coffee takes time to brew and soda is not considered a "serious" energy-enhancing beverage. Energy drinks fill the niche between caffeinated coffee and caffeinated soda, giving you an energy boost, which is code for staying awake chemically for long periods of time. These beverages contain caffeine in combination with other presumed energy-enhancing ingredients, such as taurine, B vitamins, and herbal extracts. (Though, when I see an energy drink touting an herbal substance, such as ginseng, as a primary ingredient, I grow suspicious. The actual ingredient label almost always lists water, sweetener, and caffeine as the top three ingredients.)

Unlike cola beverages, which have their caffeine levels limited by the Food and Drug Administration in the United States, energy drinks are not subject to such limitations. Most energy drinks contain about 80 milligrams of caffeine per eight-ounce serving, although some contain as much as 300 milligrams. In comparison, the same amount of tea contains around 30 milligrams of caffeine, while coffee has about 90 milligrams. To ensure consumer safety, it would seem wise to have warnings on labels of energy drinks that contain elevated levels of active ingredients, especially caffeine.[1] In addition, an acceptable upper limit should be put in place for the allowable amount of caffeine that can be put in these products. To get a better understanding of these products, let us take a look at Red Bull, the beverage that put energy drinks on the map.

RED BULL

INGREDIENTS

Carbonated water, sucrose, glucose, sodium citrate, taurine, glucuronolactone, caffeine, inositol, niacinamide, calcium pantothenate, pyridoxine HCl, Vitamin B_{12}, artificial flavors and colors.

NUTRITION FACTS (8.3 FLUID OUNCES)

Calories: 110	Sodium: 200 milligrams
Carbohydrates: 28 grams	Protein: 0
Sugar: 27 grams	Caffeine: 80 milligrams
Total Fat: 0	

OUNCE-PER-OUNCE SUGAR COUNT!

The following table ranks a number of popular beverages according to the amount of sugar contained in an eight-ounce serving. As you can see, the amount is shocking. Even more disturbing is that these and most beverages are sold in bottles and cans that hold much more than eight ounces. (See "Think Before You Drink!" on page 40.)

Beverage (8 fluid ounces)	Approximate Sugar Content in Teaspoons (4.2 grams = 1 teaspoon)
Mountain Dew Sugar: 31 grams	
Pepsi Sugar: 28 grams	
Coca-Cola Sugar: 27 grams	
SunnyD Tangy Original Sugar: 27 grams	
Red Bull Energy Drink Sugar: 26 grams	
AriZona Lemon Tea Sugar: 24 grams	
Tropicana Pure Premium Orange Juice Sugar: 22 grams	
Snapple Lemon Tea Sugar: 21 grams	
Gatorade Original Lemon-Lime Sugar: 14 grams	
Vitamin Water Essential Sugar: 13 grams	

THINK BEFORE YOU DRINK!

In the table on page 39, the following sugary beverages are compared according to the amount of sugar contained in an eight-ounce serving. Unfortunately, these drinks are sold in cans and bottles meant for individual consumption that contain much more than eight ounces. The table below shows the sugar content—as well as the calorie count and caffeine level—of the same products in their most commonly available containers.

Beverage in Popular Sizes	Approximate Sugar Content in Teaspoons (1 teaspoon = 4.2 grams)
Mountain Dew	
Category: Soft drink	
Size: **20 fluid ounces**	
Calories: 290	
Caffeine: 91 milligrams	
Sugar: 77 grams	
Pepsi	
Category: Soft drink	
Size: **20 fluid ounces**	
Calories: 250	
Caffeine: 63 milligrams	
Sugar: 69 grams	
Coca-Cola	
Category: Soft drink	
Size: **20 fluid ounces**	
Calories: 240	
Caffeine: 57 milligrams	
Sugar: 65 grams	
AriZona Lemon Tea	
Category: Iced tea	
Size: **20 fluid ounces**	
Calories: 225	
Caffeine: 37.5 milligrams	
Sugar: 60 grams	

Beverage in Popular Sizes	Approximate Sugar Content in Teaspoons (1 teaspoon = 4.2 grams)
Snapple Lemon Tea Category: Iced tea Size: **16 fluid ounces** Calories: 160 Caffeine: 42 milligrams Sugar: 42 grams	
SunnyD Tangy Original Category: Fruit drink Size: **16 fluid ounces** Calories: 180 Sugar: 40 grams	
Gatorade Original Lemon-Lime Category: Sports drink Size: **20 fluid ounces** Calories: 130 Sugar: 34 grams	
Tropicana Pure Premium Orange Juice Category: Fruit juice Size: **12 fluid ounces** Calories: 165 Sugar: 33 grams	
Vitamin Water Essential Category: Enhanced water Volume: **20 fluid ounces** Calories: 125 Sugar: 32.5 grams	
Red Bull Category: Energy drink Size: **8.3 fluid ounces** Calories: 110 Caffeine: 80 milligrams Sugar: 27 grams	

ICED TEA

Polyphenols are a type of antioxidant commonly found in tea. Antioxidants protect your cells from damage caused by free radicals. Polyphenols can actually block the actions of certain enzymes that promote cancer growth.[2] But if you think you are getting lots of polyphenols in that bottle or can of iced tea, think again. Research presented at the American Chemical Society's 240th National Meeting showed that it would take twenty bottles of black or green tea to have the same amount of polyphenols that are contained in a cup of freshly brewed green or black tea.

Besides the plain black and green teas that come in bottles, you would be amazed at all the new flavored black and green teas now on the market. Most use sugar, high-fructose corn syrup, or a sugar substitute as a sweetener. The Tazo Tea Company's Giant Peach Iced Tea drink is a prime example. It seems harmless, but once you've drunk a whole bottle, you've ingested a lot of sugar.

TAZO GIANT PEACH ICED TEA

INGREDIENTS
An infusion of (water, green teas), organic cane sugar, concentrated apple juice, natural peach flavor, concentrated peach juice, ginger juice, citric acid, and concentrated elderberry juice.

NUTRITION FACTS (13.8 FLUID OUNCES)

Calories: 160	Total Fat: 0
Carbohydrates: 36 grams	Sodium: 15 milligrams
Sugar: 35 grams	Protein: 0

FRUIT JUICE

It does not matter if you squeeze it from fresh fruit, get it from a bottle or can, or reconstruct it from concentrate, real fruit juice— no matter which brand you choose—will always contain the same amount of sugar and calories. In order to drink an eight-ounce glass of fresh orange juice, you would need to consume at least four oranges, depending on their size, which is unlikely. It is far better, however, to peel and eat one orange than it is to drink a glass of orange juice. Because fruit juice lacks many of the important digestive elements present in whole fruit, such as fiber, a glass of fresh fruit juice will elevate your blood sugar far more rapidly than an actual piece of fruit. *And while you might reach for a glass of OJ for an easy dose of vitamin C, the truth is that the high sugar content of the juice actually disrupts the metabolism of vitamins, making them much less effective.* In reality, when it comes to sugar content, if you drink a glass of Tropicana Pure Premium Orange Juice every day, you might as well be drinking a glass of soda, as you can see from the following information.

TROPICANA PURE PREMIUM ORANGE JUICE

INGREDIENTS

100 percent orange juice.

NUTRITION FACTS (8 FLUID OUNCES)

Calories: 110	Calcium: 2% Daily Value
Carbohydrates: 26 grams	Thiamin: 10% Daily Value
Sugar: 22 grams	Riboflavin: 4% Daily Value
Total Fat: 0	Niacin: 4% Daily Value
Sodium: 0	Vitamin B_6: 6% Daily Value
Potassium: 450 milligrams	Folic Acid: 15% Daily Value
Protein: 2 grams	Magnesium: 6% Daily Value
	Vitamin C: 120% Daily Value

FRUIT DRINKS

A fruit drink is a sweetened beverage of diluted fruit juice. Unlike fruit juices, which contain 100 percent actual juice, fruit drinks are composed of a smaller percentage of juice (in many cases, just 5 percent), as well as sweetener and other possible additives. For example, lemonade, Hi-C, and Kool-Aid are considered fruit drinks because they offer only a limited amount of actual juice and have added sugar. Just one look at the ingredients of Hawaiian Punch Fruit Juicy Red will tell you how truly limited this type of beverage is in its content of actual juice. *In addition, even if these beverages contain vitamins, do not be fooled into thinking they are at all healthful. As you know, sugary drinks disturb your body's ability to absorb these important nutrients.*

HAWAIIAN PUNCH FRUIT JUICY RED

INGREDIENTS

Water, high fructose corn syrup, and 2% or less of each of the following: concentrated juices (pineapple, orange, passion fruit and apple), purees (apricot, papaya, guava), citric acid, natural and artificial flavors, pectin, gum acacia, gum ghatti, glycerol ester of wood rosin, sodium hexametaphosphate, red #40, blue #1, sodium benzoate and potassium sorbate (preservatives) and ascorbic acid (vitamin C).

NUTRITION FACTS (20 FLUID OUNCES)

Calories: 300	Sodium: 300 milligrams
Carbohydrates: 75 grams	Protein: 0
Sugar: 70 grams	Vitamin C: 250% Daily Value
Total Fat: 0	

ENHANCED WATER

Enhanced water is simply water with added vitamins, minerals, electrolytes, herbs, and other possible substances. Although there may be healthful ingredients in the water, just check the label. *After water, the next ingredient on the list is often sugar or another type of sweetener, which interferes with any potential benefit that may be had from the aforementioned "enhancements."* Some enhanced water products even contain caffeine. Trying to pose as a healthful drink with flavors named "Energy," "Defense," and "Revive," Glacéau Vitamin Water is really just sugar water produced by the Coca-Cola Company, not to mention one of the most popular drinks in this category.

GLACÉAU VITAMIN WATER ESSENTIAL

INGREDIENTS

Reverse osmosis water, crystalline fructose, cane sugar, less than 0.5% of: citric acid, potassium phosphate (electrolyte), natural flavor, vitamin C (ascorbic acid), calcium lactate (electrolyte), gum acacia, magnesium lactate (electrolyte), vitamin B_3 (niacinamide), vitamin E (alpha-tocopheryl acetate), vitamin B_5 (calcium pantothenate), glycerol ester of rosin, vitamin B_6 (pyridoxine hydrochloride), Vitamin B_{12}, beta-carotene, modified food starch, sorbitol.

NUTRITION FACTS (20 FLUID OUNCES)

Calories: 125

Carbohydrates: 32.5 grams

Sugar: 32.5 grams

Total fat: 0

Sodium: 0

Potassium: 175 milligrams

Protein: 0

Vitamin A: 25% Daily Value

Vitamin B_3: 100% Daily Value

Vitamin B_5: 100% Daily Value

Vitamin B_6: 100% Daily Value

Vitamin B_{12}: 100% Daily Value

Vitamin C: 300% Daily Value

Vitamin E: 25% Daily Value

Calcium: 10% Daily Value

COCKTAIL MIXERS

Cocktail mixers come in a wide variety of flavors and are combined with alcohol to make mixed drinks. Since these mixers are rarely used without alcohol, I will not discuss them at great length in this book, but I will say that there is often quite a lot of sugar or high-fructose corn syrup in these products, so read the labels carefully. Just two tablespoons of Rose's Grenadine, which adds a pomegranate flavor to cocktails, also adds an astounding amount of sugar to the drink, as the following information reveals.

ROSE'S GRENADINE

INGREDIENTS

High-fructose corn syrup, water, citric acid, natural and artificial flavors, sodium citrate, sodium benzoate, red 40, blue 1.

NUTRITION FACTS (2 TABLESPOONS)

Calories: 90	Total Fat: 0
Carbohydrates: 22 grams	Sodium: 10 milligrams
Sugar: 21 grams	Protein: 0

MEAL SUPPLEMENT DRINKS FOR ADULTS

Meal replacement beverages are designed to promote weight gain, and are generally used by those who may have trouble maintaining a healthful weight, such as the elderly or the ill. Of the many brands of meal replacements, Ensure is definitely one of the most popular. But check the label of Ensure's Nutrition Shake and you may get scared. The first four ingredients are water, corn maltodextrin, sugar (sucrose), and corn syrup. So what exactly is corn maltodextrin?

Maltodextrin, as explained in Chapter 3, is a complex carbohydrate used to add sweetness and a smooth texture to drinks. It allows manufacturers to add less sugar to their beverages without making them any less sweet. Because it is not technically a sugar, manufacturers can then state "no sugar" or "low sugar" on the nutrition label of a drink that contains maltodextrin. For example, Ensure's label lists only 18 grams of sugar. But don't be fooled. It also lists 41 grams of carbohydrates, which consist of the 18 grams of sugar previously mentioned along with 23 grams of maltodextrin. This number may still seem reasonable, but the fact is that maltodextrin actually raises blood sugar higher than do high-fructose corn syrup, sucrose, and glucose.

Ensure doesn't consider maltodextrin a sugar, but I do. In my opinion, every eight-ounce serving of Ensure has 41 grams of sugar, and that is a lot more than a Coke of the same size. *While it may be true that Ensure has lots of vitamins and minerals, the sugar it contains will upset your body chemistry so that your cells won't be able to absorb these nutrients properly.*

ENSURE NUTRITION SHAKE

INGREDIENTS

Water, corn maltodextrin, sugar (sucrose), corn syrup, milk protein concentrate, cocoa powder (processed with alkali), soy oil, soy protein isolate, canola oil, vitamins, and minerals.

NUTRITION FACTS (8 FLUID OUNCES)

Calories: 250

Carbohydrates: 41 grams

Sugar: 18 grams

Total Fat: 6 grams

Sodium: 200 milligrams

Potassium: 420 milligrams

Protein: 9 grams

MEAL SUPPLEMENT DRINKS FOR CHILDREN

In addition to the meal supplements for adults, there are also versions for children. They are meant to provide the necessary nutrients for proper growth and development to infants and young children who may be too picky to eat a well-balanced diet. These products come in different flavors, including chocolate. (I am not sure why a child needs a chocolate drink.) One of the most popular brands of meal replacements is Pediasure. As is the case with Ensure, the first three ingredients of Pediasure are frightening. They include water, sucrose, and corn maltodextrin. The label says that eight ounces of Pediasure contain 23 grams of sugar and 31 grams of carbohydrates. Aside from sugar, the only other ingredient that could be classified as a carbohydrate is maltodextrin, with its high glycemic index. Therefore, because I consider maltodextrin a sugar, the actual sugar content in this children's drink is 31 grams, which, again, is more than a Coke of the same size. I am just giving you the facts. You can draw your own conclusions. But remember, this is a product meant for children.

PEDIASURE CHOCOLATE

INGREDIENTS

Water, sugar (sucrose), corn maltodextrin, milk protein concentrate, high-oleic safflower oil, soy oil, cocoa powder (processed with alkali), soy protein isolate, medium-chain triglycerides, vitamins, and minerals.

NUTRITION FACTS (8 FLUID OUNCES)

Calories: 240

Carbohydrates: 31 grams

Sugar: 23 grams

Protein: 7 grams

Total Fat: 9 grams

Sodium: 90 milligrams

Potassium: 310 milligrams

CONCLUSION

No matter which drink you choose, it is always important to recognize the size of one serving. Remember that these beverages come in cartons, cans, or bottles that range from eight to eighty-nine ounces, and sometimes more. But that carton, can, or bottle does not usually represent just one serving. Typically, one serving size will be listed as eight or twelve ounces. Therefore, if you drink a whole container of any beverage, you could be getting two or more times the amount of sugar, caffeine, and other questionable ingredients stated on the label. The harm comes mostly from the sugar and sweeteners, but some of those other additives are equally scary.

Now that you know a little more about the different types of sugary drinks that have become so common in our culture, it is time to discuss the many diseases that have been connected to their consumption.

5

Links to Current Health Epidemics

While researching numerous journal articles in preparation for this book, even I was shocked at how many different sugary drinks could be linked to disease. Moreover, it was virtually impossible to find any redeeming nutritional value to soda or sweetened beverages. They do not promote healthful nourishment and offer nothing more than empty calories. It seems as though their main role is to upset body chemistry, resulting in sickness. The length of this text does not allow me to highlight all of the many possible connections between illness and the varied ingredients contained in sodas and other sweetened drinks, so I will focus on the three most lethal substances found in these products: sugar (and sugar substitutes), caffeine, and phosphoric acid, which were detailed in Chapter 3. By the time you finish reading about the many dangerous health conditions related to soda and other sweetened beverages, I suspect you will decide to reduce your intake of these drinks significantly or cut them out of your life completely.

ACID REFLUX AND ABDOMINAL DISCOMFORT

The phosphoric acid and carbon dioxide in soft drinks have been associated with a process known as *acid reflux*, in which digestive acids splash out of your stomach and into your esophagus, often causing a burning sensation in your chest. This condition is commonly called *heartburn*.[1] In addition, fructose has been known to cause impaired digestion and gas, resulting in belching, flatulence, abdominal bloating, and abdominal pain. Unfortunately, most people might not recognize soda's role in these problems, as symptoms may not show up until a few hours after consuming a soft drink.[2]

ASTHMA AND ALLERGIES

Having trouble breathing? Can't live without an inhaler? Many food additives can make asthma worse and may even cause the condition in the first place. Scientists have found that sodium benzoate, a preservative found in soft drinks, can actually cause asthma episodes[3] and recommend that asthma sufferers avoid it.[4] In addition to sodium benzoate, sugar also seems to be a possible trigger of asthma attacks. In a study conducted on mice, the consumption of sugar water resulted in more than twice as much airway inflammation than the consumption of plain water. The sugar seemed to make the mice that were fed sugar water more prone to the condition.[5]

Another problem that sodium benzoate can cause is an allergic reaction called *anaphylaxis.* Unlike most allergic reactions, however, anaphylaxis is life-threatening. It occurs almost immediately upon exposure to an allergen and includes symptoms such as itchiness, palpitations, light-headedness, difficulty swallowing, and difficulty breathing. The most severe cases of anaphylaxis result in complete closure of the airways, shock, and death.[6]

Although research has made connections between some of the ingredients in soda and a few allergies, I believe that further study will uncover links between soft drinks and many other types of allergies.

CANCER

The link between cancer and the sugar found in soda has long been established. In 1927, Otto Warburg published a Nobel Prize-winning paper that explained the way in which cancer tumors actually feed off sugar, a process referred to as fermentation.[7] These days, doctors use this process to detect cancer, finding the source of the disease by administering radioactive glucose, which finds its way to the tumor and causes the growth to show up on a scan.[8]

Of all forms of cancer, pancreatic cancer seems to be the most studied in correlation with the consumption of sugar and soda. Perhaps this is because diabetes, a disease that affects your body's ability to metabolize sugar, is the result of an improperly functioning pancreas. It stands to reason that sugar might also lead to cancer in the same organ. But who gets diabetes, who gets pancreatic cancer, and who gets both? Those answers are buried in genetics. However, by avoiding soft drinks and other sugary beverages, you are less likely to have to worry about the illnesses that may be lurking in your genes.

In a study performed in Sweden, food questionnaires were filled out by nearly 80,000 men and women whose health statuses were followed over the next seven years. Consumption of added sugar, soft drinks, and sweetened fruit soups or stewed fruit proved to be strongly associated with the cases of pancreatic cancer that developed. In fact, while sugar showed a connection to a high risk of pancreatic cancer, soda was linked to an even higher chance of getting the disease. These results suggest that it is more than just the sugar in soda that causes the illness.[9] There is something else going on that we have yet to understand.

There is admittedly quite a bit of variance from study to study concerning soft drinks and pancreatic cancer, but they all paint soda as a cancer-causing menace. For example, according to one study, sugar was found to have a greater carcinogenic effect on men than women, and low-calorie diet soda was actually found to be more to blame for pancreatic cancer than regular soda.[10] In a Harvard University study of the pancreatic cancer risk of subjects with a history of diabetes, women who consumed a high amount of sugar-sweetened soft drinks seemed to put themselves more at risk of pancreatic cancer than men in the same category.[11]

Furthermore, a health study of soda and juice consumption conducted in Singapore found that drinking two sodas per week created an elevated risk of pancreatic cancer for both men and women.[12] Finally, researchers in Los Angeles discovered that pancreatic cancer patients had significantly higher fasting blood fructose levels than non-cancer patients.[13]

In reference to other forms of the disease, a diet that includes soda and other forms of sugar has been connected to an increased risk of gastric cancer,[14] while blood glucose levels have been associated with the prognosis of ovarian cancer.[15] In a study out of England, researchers linked colorectal, ovarian, and breast cancer to increased consumption of various types of sugar, including sucrose, while also discovering that dietary fiber reduces colorectal cancer risk.[16]

As you can see, there seems to be an interesting trend in the types of cancer that have been directly associated with soda and other sugary drinks. It appears that pancreatic, gastric, and colorectal cancer in particular have a strong connection to soft drink consumption, but forms such as lung and laryngeal cancer do not. But whatever the main cause of a cancer happens to be, I would argue that soda creates favorable conditions for the disease to flourish in general. For example, results of a study in Belgium showed a positive correlation between the amount of soda ingested by girls during puberty and breast cancer risk.[17] Soda may not cause breast cancer directly, but it certainly seems to give the illness the right environment to occur in the future.

CARDIOVASCULAR DISEASE

According to a statement made by the American Heart Association (AHA) regarding dietary sugar intake and heart disease, the safe upper limit of daily added sugar is no more than 100 calories for women and 150 calories for men. These amounts translate to six teaspoons of sugar for women and nine for men.[18, 19] Amazingly, these limits require a 70-percent reduction in the current average level of sugar consumption. In light of this information

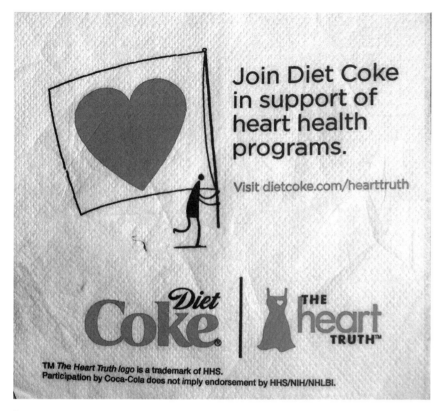

Join Diet Coke
in support of
heart health
programs.

Visit dietcoke.com/hearttruth

Diet Coke

THE heart TRUTH™

TM *The Heart Truth logo* is a trademark of HHS.
Participation by Coca-Cola does not imply endorsement by HHS/NIH/NHLBI.

This Diet Coke ad, shown here on an airplane napkin, attempts to link the soda with the government's "Heart Truth" campaign against heart disease. The ad suggests that Diet Coke is a healthful alternative to regular soda. The truth, however, is in the fine print, which states that this point of view is not endorsed by any of the health groups behind the campaign.

and without taking into consideration all other sources of sugar in your diet, drinking one sugar-sweetened soda every day is enough to put you at risk of heart disease, as there are approximately ten teaspoons of sugar in one twelve-ounce can.

In 2001, the Department of Health and Human Services began a campaign to raise awareness of heart disease in women called "The Heart Truth." The Coca-Cola Company showed support for the cause by marketing Diet Coke in connection with the organization.20 Both Coca-Cola and The Heart Truth promoted the idea of diet soft drinks as a safe alternative to regular soda, advertising it in a variety of places, from websites to paper napkins on airplanes. And although The Heart Truth campaign did not endorse Diet Coke outright, both logos were featured together prominently. It was a sneaky bit of advertising on the part of the Coca-Cola Company, which hoped no one would read the fine print.

Unfortunately, research that followed more than 2,500 New Yorkers for nine or more years has a different story to tell about diet soda. According to a recent presentation given at the American Stroke Association's International Stroke Conference in Los Angeles, subjects who drank diet soda every day increased their chance of experiencing a cardiovascular event such as a heart attack or stroke by 61 percent over those who did not consume soft drinks. Whether this increased risk was caused by an ingredient in diet soda or some other factor that diet soda drinkers seem to have in common is still unknown. Regardless, the information is worthy of your attention, as it marks the first time that diet soda consumption has been associated with an elevated risk of stroke and other cardiovascular problems. Artificial sweeteners, however, have been associated with many other health complications, so these findings are not surprising.

EPILEPSY, MENTAL HEALTH, TOURETTE SYNDROME, HEADACHES

Soft drinks and similar sweetened beverages can affect your brain and mental health in alarming ways. Cases have been reported of individuals who experienced mild seizures after heavy consumption of energy drinks such as Red Bull. Furthermore, the episodes seemed to clear up once the subjects stopped drinking these products.[21] In addition, a Norwegian study found that teenagers who drank an average of four sodas per day displayed a high degree of mental health problems, including anxiety, dizziness, hopelessness, sadness, sleeplessness, and unhappiness.[22] Finally, the aspartame and sucralose used to sweeten diet drinks have been linked to headaches in certain people.[23]

Caffeinated soft drinks have also been associated with an increase in the number of tics experienced by sufferers of Tourette syndrome.[24] In fact, one teenage boy who had endured tics since the age of seven saw all of his Tourette syndrome symptoms disappear after six months of avoiding all caffeinated beverages and foods. The symptoms, however, returned once caffeine was reintroduced into his diet. Similar results were shown in connection with the subject's cousin as well.[25]

GOUT

When the level of uric acid in your blood becomes elevated, it often crystallizes and collects in your joints and tendons, causing repeated bouts of inflammation. This condition is called *gout* and has been linked to certain dietary habits such as fructose consumption. Sugar-sweetened beverages that include soft drinks, sports drinks, and fruit juices are a common source of fructose and have been shown to raise uric acid levels. Studies have suggested that five to six servings of sugar-sweetened drinks per week can significantly increase your chance of developing gout. Research has also shown that men who consume two or more servings of sugar-sweetened soft drinks each day have an 85-percent greater chance of gout than men who ingest less than one serving per week.[26, 27] And though the condition is most common in men over forty, uric acid levels can spike even in teenagers.

HYPERTENSION

Hypertension, also known as high blood pressure, is another aspect of the metabolic syndrome that has been linked to soda consumption. In separate studies, both caffeine and high-fructose corn syrup were shown to contribute to hypertension. Moreover, the study on caffeine made no distinction between regular and diet soda.[28] Both drinks were associated with high blood pressure. Frighteningly, the study on high-fructose corn syrup actually suggested a relationship between the sweetener and *all* aspects of the metabolic syndrome, not just hypertension.[29]

31 Ways Soft Drinks and Other Sweetened Beverages Can Ruin Your Health

The consumption of soda and other sugary beverages can lead to a variety of health problems. Compiled from information published in medical journals and scientific publications, and found on health and medical websites, the following list features some of the many ways in which your soft drink habit can seriously compromise your well-being.

1. Sweetened beverages can cause weight gain, leading to obesity.

2. Drinking two sugar-sweetened soft drinks a day may lead to long-term liver damage.

3. Caffeinated soft drinks have been linked to mood swings.

4. Soft drinks can cause inflammation in your body.

5. Sugar-sweetened soft drinks stress your body's ability to process sugar, possibly leading to diabetes.

6. By drinking sugar-sweetened soft drinks, you may increase your blood pressure, your risk of developing hypertension, and your risk of cardiovascular disease.

7. The acidity of soft drinks dissolves tooth enamel.

8. Cola consumption has been linked to osteoporosis in women.

9. The fructose in sugary drinks has been associated with an increased risk of gout.

10. Consumption of crystalline fructose may result in mild gastrointestinal distress.

11. Cola has been linked to caffeine headaches in children.

12. Cola can decrease high-density lipoproteins (HDL), otherwise known as "good" cholesterol.

13. Soft drinks have been implicated in the development of the metabolic syndrome. (See page 58.)

14. The caffeine, sugar, and artificial sweeteners found in beverages can result in addiction.

15. Artificial sweeteners can trigger bladder contractions, leading to incontinence.

16. By drinking two or more soft drinks per week, you increase your risk of pancreatic cancer by nearly double.

17. The acidity of soft drinks can leach calcium from your bones.

18. Diet soft drinks increase the risk of preterm delivery in pregnant women.

19. Caffeinated soft drinks may promote tics in susceptible children.

20. Sugar-sweetened colas have been linked to a high risk of gestational diabetes.

21. Excessive cola consumption can lead to low potassium levels, also known as *hypokalemia,* leading to muscle weakness and possible paralysis.

22. Fructose intake may impair memory.

23. Soft drinks can cause the development of kidney stones.

24. Soft drinks can lead to reduced sperm concentration and a lower total sperm count.

25. Caffeinated drinks may lead to symptoms of depression in adolescents.

26. Elevated soda consumption has been associated with epilepsy.

27. Prepubescent girls who drink soda have been shown to begin menstruation at an earlier age than normal, which may lead to breast cancer later in life.

28. Adolescents who drink sugar-sweetened beverages on a regular basis have high uric acid levels.

29. Cola drinks can stain your teeth yellow.

30. Soda has been linked to cancer of the esophagus.

31. The consumption of one can of soda results in 53.5 minutes of elevated stomach acid.

* Citations for the entries in this inset are found on page 116 of the References.

HYPOKALEMIA

Hypokalemia is defined by a low level of potassium in your blood, which typically leads to muscular weakness. This condition has been associated with the consumption of cola-based soft drinks—in particular, the glucose, fructose, and caffeine contained in these beverages. Studies have shown that even frequent cola drinkers can improve the symptoms of hypokalemia by cutting back on the number of soft drinks they have.[30]

THE METABOLIC SYNDROME

The metabolic syndrome consists of a number of health conditions that, when occurring simultaneously, predict the onset of diabetes and cardiovascular disease. These conditions generally include elevated waist circumference, raised fasting blood glucose, high LDL cholesterol, low HDL cholesterol, raised triglycerides, and elevated blood pressure. The troublesome reality is that soda is linked to all aspects of the metabolic syndrome. In the same way that sugar, caffeine, and phosphoric acid work together to acidify the body and promote bone loss and tooth decay, these ingredients can ultimately lead to one or more of the above-mentioned conditions. In particular, soft drink consumption has been directly related to higher incidences of these risk factors in middle-aged adults.[31]

NON-ALCOHOLIC FATTY LIVER DISEASE

Non-alcoholic liver disease is defined by the buildup of fat in your liver that cannot be attributed to alcohol consumption. Researchers have discovered that soda increases your risk of non-alcoholic fatty liver disease regardless of whether you show symptoms of the metabolic syndrome or not.[32]

OBESITY

Soft drinks promote weight gain in two ways. They not only add harmful ingredients to your diet but also tend to replace healthful foods, such as fruits and vegetables.[33] Fruits and vegetables contain fiber, which helps prevent your body from converting sugar into fat. Basically, soft drinks put sugar in your body without the addition of any helpful substances that might lessen the sweetener's damaging effects.

According to research connecting adolescent obesity and fast-food restaurants, subjects who drank more soda than their peers also consumed fewer fruits and vegetables, and were more likely to be overweight or obese.[34] In addition, a study that sampled 200 children of the Cree Indian tribe, whose diet largely consisted of energy-dense but nutrient-poor foods such as sweetened beverages, found that 64 percent of its subjects were either overweight or obese. Furthermore, 98 percent of the children in the study reported eating less than five fruits and vegetables per day.[35] In another study, adults who sporadically drank soda were 15 percent more likely to be overweight or obese compared to those who did not include soft drinks in their diet. In addition, adults who drank at least one soft drink per day were 27 percent more likely to be obese.[36]

High-fructose corn syrup, the main sweetener in soft drinks, was shown to increase obesity levels significantly more than sucrose in a study conducted on rats.[37] As cited by the researchers, fructose is metabolized by the liver into fat, raising triglycerides and leading to insulin resistance. It also suppresses the hormone *leptin,* which lets your body know when it is full, causing you to eat even when you are no longer actually hungry. Diets high in fructose, therefore, increase the likelihood of not only weight gain but also a number of other aspects of the metabolic syndrome.[38] We should all be concerned by the drastic increase in HFCS consumption that has occurred over the last forty years.[39]

Unfortunately, artificial sweeteners don't reduce your risk of obesity or any other element of the metabolic syndrome. In fact, in some cases, researchers have found that they pose a greater risk than regular sugar in terms of promoting fat deposits and high blood pressure.[40] Ultimately, whether a soft drink contains artificial sweetener or a sugar-based product, it will lead you down the road to weight gain and possible obesity. And, as you now know, the link between obesity and illness is well established. By consuming sugar-sweetened beverages instead of more healthful choices, such as plain water, you increase your chances of acquiring diabetes and cardiovascular disease.[41]

REPRODUCTIVE PROBLEMS

In a Danish study that looked at the relationship between caffeine intake and semen quality, high levels of caffeine from cola consumption were found to decrease semen quality more than did comparable levels of caffeine from other sources such as coffee. Researchers suggested that while caffeine had a negative effect on semen quality, other additives contained in soda seemed to worsen the effect even further.[42] I would think that sugar might be the main culprit.

In another Danish study, which involved pregnant women, an association was made between the intake of artificially sweetened soft drinks and an increased risk of preterm delivery. No association was observed between sugar-sweetened soft drinks and pregnancy, [43] but this fact doesn't mean that a pregnant woman should drink sugar-sweetened soda. Truly, the best idea for a pregnant woman is to keep her body in a constant state of homeostasis, which will help ensure the delivery of a healthy baby. As sugar upsets homeostasis, I recommend that pregnant women avoid soft drinks and any other sweetened beverages, whether natural or artificial.

TOOTH DECAY AND OSTEOPOROSIS

Sugar, caffeine, and phosphoric acid all rot your teeth and soften your bones. All three ingredients create a witch's brew that can cause dental caries, also known as *cavities*, and bone loss, also known as *osteoporosis*. While I have put tooth decay and bone loss into the same category, the soda industry has conceded an association between its products and tooth decay only. They have not admitted a connection to osteoporosis or any other disease for that matter. Tooth decay and bone loss, however, are similar processes in which the hard structures of teeth and bones are softened through demineralization, rendering them susceptible to breakage and rot.

When you consume the sugar, caffeine, and phosphoric acid contained in a soft drink, you throw your body out of homeostasis, making it more acidic than it should be. As discussed in Chapter 1, when your system becomes acidic, it pulls calcium from your bones to bring itself back into balance. Unfortunately, when your body is finished with this process, it cannot put the excess calcium back into your bones. Instead, the calcium can build up in your system, causing arthritis, dental plaque, and bone spurs, or it is excreted from the body through the urine.

Dentists have linked soft drink consumption to dental caries for decades now. Completed in 1974, government-funded studies proved a direct link between tooth decay and soft drinks.[44] In 1994, these findings were reconfirmed and expanded to assert that the effects were cumulative.[45] In fact, soft drinks continue to be implicated in tooth decay. According to research, children who consume soda develop cavities almost twice as often as those who drink milk or pure fruit juice.[46] This is likely because soda works a triple whammy on teeth. First, it acidifies your system, contributing to demineralization, as mentioned above. Second, the sugar changes the chemical composition of saliva so that it can no longer flush away the bacteria that can cause cavities. Third, the bacteria eat the sugar, producing acids that erode tooth enamel, which has been weakened by demineralization. While sugar is the main factor behind tooth decay, caffeine and phosphoric acid certainly speed the process.

Despite what soft drink companies would have you believe, soda not only rots your teeth but also softens your bones. Research has linked the consumption of soda to a higher risk of obesity, decreased calcium levels, and increased urinary calcium excretion, all of which sets the stage for osteoporosis later in life.[47] Colas have also been implicated in the reduction of bone mineral density in women.[48] In one study, caffeine and phosphoric acid were shown to limit calcium absorption. Though the study did not take into account the role of sugar in bone loss, its results spelled it out plainly. Subjects with a high intake of regular cola (containing caffeine, phosphoric acid, and sugar) had elevated bone loss, while drinkers of diet cola (caffeine, phosphoric acid, and artificial sweetener) had slightly less damage. As you might suspect, those who did not drink colas at all had the least amount of bone loss.

In particular, there is great concern for adolescent girls who drink cola regularly, as some research suggests that they break bones five times as often as those who do not consume the beverage. Scientists feel that colas consumed during peak periods of bone growth, such as adolescence, heighten the problem.[49] Your teeth and bones are the hardest tissues in your body. If sugar destroys your teeth and weakens your bones, just imagine what it does to the soft tissues in your body, such as your kidneys, liver, and heart.

Although this book primarily deals with the dangers of soft drinks, when it comes to bone loss, coffee is also a culprit. Caffeine is specifically listed as an osteoporosis-causing agent in numerous studies regarding excessive coffee consumption. In fact, lifetime usage of caffeinated coffee equal to two cups per day has been connected to a significant decrease in women's overall bone mineral density.[50]

TYPE 2 DIABETES

Type 2 diabetes is essentially the failure of your body to metabolize sugar. Unlike type 1 diabetes, in which the body produces insufficient insulin, this disease occurs when cells become resistant to the hormone. Both of these possibilities can occur from eating too much sugar over a long period of time. And as you know, soft drinks are one of the biggest sources of sugar in the average diet. While sugar is the ingredient that is most closely linked to diabetes, it is not the only ingredient in soda that can lead to the disease.

Because fructose does not trigger the production of insulin, the soda industry often states that high-fructose corn syrup is actually better for diabetics than regular table sugar. High-fructose corn syrup, as you learned earlier in the book, is made up of 55 percent fructose, while table sugar comprises 50 percent fructose. Fructose may not raise blood sugar levels, but this doesn't mean that it cannot cause diabetes. In one study, rats that consumed fructose developed type 2 diabetes at least two months earlier than rats that were fed table sugar.[51] This result was most likely due to excess triglycerides (fat in the blood) caused by fructose consumption. Some researchers feel that excess triglycerides increase the chance of insulin resistance, essentially finding a way through the back door to cause diabetes without the help of increased sugar intake.

In addition, researchers have long noticed that caffeine stimulates the pancreas in similar ways to glucose and sucrose. Specifically, it promotes the production of "fight or flight" hormones called *catecholamines,* which are released by your adrenal glands in response to stress. In other words, caffeine has the same effect on your body as stress. It makes your heart pump faster and your liver release stored sugar, raising your blood sugar level and resulting in the secretion of insulin by your pancreas.[52] In one study, caffeine ingestion was shown to contribute to insulin resistance in both obese men and men of normal weight.[53]

Unfortunately, children and pregnant women are also being affected by this plague. In a study conducted on gestational diabetes, which occurs only during pregnancy, drinking soda five times a week was shown to increase the onset of the disease by 22 percent. Gestational diabetes is a major complication of pregnancy and sometimes leads to full-blown type 2 diabetes.[54] In another study conducted on adolescents, researchers concluded that both the removal of sugar equivalent to one can of soda and the addition of fiber equivalent to one cup of beans per day led to significant reductions in the risk of type 2 diabetes.[55] Imagine if adolescents stopped drinking soda *and* ate more fiber!

And if you think that simply switching to diet soda will eliminate your chance of acquiring diabetes, think again. In one study, twenty-two healthy volunteers had their blood glucose levels tested after drinking equivalent amounts of diet soda or carbonated water. While neither drink put more glucose into the blood stream than the other, diet soda consumption was associated with higher insulin secretion. This suggests that even diet soda, which does not contain glucose, can contribute to pancreatic exertion, one aspect of type 2 diabetes.[56]

While I'm sure that other substances in soda can be linked to this disease, research on ingredients other than sugar and caffeine may be hard to perform, as many of these substances appear only in combination with sugar and caffeine, making it hard to determine which chemical caused which result. To stay healthy, the best form of soda to drink is truly none at all.

URINARY STONES, KIDNEY STONES, KIDNEY DISEASE, AND OVERACTIVE BLADDER

As described in Chapter 1, when your body becomes too acidic, it pulls calcium from your bones to regain its internal balance. This reaction can sometimes create an excess of calcium in your blood, which may then result in the formation of small calcium stones in your bladder, known as *urinary stones,* or in your kidneys, known as *kidney stones.* Soda consumption—and the phosphoric acid in soda, in particular—has been linked to these various stones. This same process also damages kidneys in other ways, leading to chronic kidney disease, which refers to the slow loss of kidney function over time. According to two studies that were conducted more than fifteen years apart, the consumption of more than two sodas a day—an amount easily met by most soda drinkers—increases your risk of both kidney stones and kidney disease.[57,58]

In connection with the artificial sweeteners found in soft drinks, a study published in *Toxicology and Applied Pharmacology* showed that acesulfame K, aspartame, and saccharin caused an enhancement in muscle contractions in the bladders of rat test subjects. In light of their findings, researchers stated that low concentrations of artificial sweeteners may be connected to the symptoms of an overactive bladder, which include the feeling of urinary urgency, increased frequency of urination, and even bouts of urinary incontinence.[59]

CONCLUSION

The illnesses that have been linked to soft drink consumption are many and varied. Whether the result of one ingredient or a combination of ingredients in soda, these diseases include everything from asthma, kidney stones, decreased semen quality, low potassium levels, and poor mental health to hypertension, heart disease, type 2 diabetes, and even cancer. More and more research exposes the ill effects of soft drinks and other sweetened beverages every day. And while the exact reason behind the association between the products and disease is at times unclear, there is an easy way to test the theory. Stop drinking the stuff and see what happens. I truly believe you will feel better. I also believe that you will improve your immunity against disease more than you may ever realize.

6

Soft Drink Addiction

It is hard to believe that a person could become addicted to regular or diet soda, or any other sweetened beverage, but it happens every day. Soft drink addiction occurs like any other. You begin by drinking one or two sodas a week, building a craving for them. Pretty soon, you find yourself wanting one or two sodas every day. Before you realize it, you need to have a soft drink in order to feel well at all. If you don't get your soda fix, you start to have symptoms of withdrawal, as you would with any addictive drug. You manage to quit the habit, but one night you decide to treat yourself to a soft drink only to get hooked again. It is a vicious cycle that could be applied to cocaine or heroin just as easily as soda.

Soft drink addiction is particularly powerful because it combines the physiological desire for caffeine and sugar with a multisensory experience that soon becomes a source of psychological comfort. You hear the unmistakable crackle of opening a soda can followed by the light fizzy sound of carbonated bubbles popping and immediately relax. This good feeling makes you take a sip of the beverage while the caffeine and sweetener then do the rest. It isn't long before you are yearning to recreate the ritual numerous times a day. As noted by Mike Adams in his book *The Five Soft*

Drink Monsters, there are many sensory components working to get you hooked on soda, including:[1]

- The feeling of wrapping your hand around a cold soft drink can or bottle.
- The distinct snap of opening a carbonated beverage.
- The clinking of ice cubes in a glass of soda.
- The tingling of the carbonation on your tongue.
- The intense sweetness of taste.
- The cool sensation in your mouth and throat.
- The sound of gulping a soft drink.

If you identify strongly with the aspects mentioned above, you may, in fact, be a soft drink addict. The simple action of lifting a container of soda to your mouth, tilting your head back, and swallowing combined with the addictive properties of these beverages is enough to be habit-forming. Found in a large number of soft drinks, the following ingredients are the ones most responsible for getting you hooked.

CAFFEINE

Soda manufacturers seem to have the same casual relationship to the truth as politicians and tobacco executives. My research for this chapter actually led me to an interesting lie. Apparently, soda manufacturers consider caffeine an integral part of many of their soft drinks when it comes to flavor. According to them—and despite caffeine being a known nerve agitator and addictive stimulant—the formulas of their flagship drinks simply cannot be changed to avoid the additive because those beverages would not taste the same without it. Of course, all of the major soda producers offer caffeine-free versions of their most popular products, so the work has actually already been done. In fact, a Johns Hopkins University study proved how off-the-wall silly the use of caffeine as a flavoring agent really is. Only 8 percent of the study's participants could tell the difference between regular soda and its caffeine-free variation.[2]

So, in light of the results of the above-mentioned study, why do soda corporations continue to include caffeine in their drinks? It would seem to me that caffeine is being used for its addictive properties, plain and simple. The more addictive a drink is, the more people will consume it, and the better the manufacturer's bottom line will look to shareholders. But caffeine isn't the only addictive substance being harnessed for profit. While you may not realize it, sweeteners are also responsible for creating and feeding the soft drink habit.

SWEETENERS

Whether it is sugar or an artificial sugar substitute such as aspartame, the sweetener in soft drinks can be addictive.[3,4] Research has shown that sugar can cause neurochemical changes in the brain similar to those that result from the use of habit-forming narcotics. Sugar consumption initiates the release of a neurotransmitter called *dopamine,* which is responsible for creating feelings of happiness and pleasure. When you binge on sugar, you produce large amounts of dopamine and soon grow accustomed to these levels. Much like caffeine addiction, once the effect of sugar wears off, you require more sugar simply to feel normal again, and experience symptoms of withdrawal if you don't get any. The reduced dopamine levels in your body make you feel depressed and unmotivated.

As you have learned earlier in this book, using artificial sweeteners is rarely a solution to the problems caused by sugar. In the case of soda addiction, it is no answer at all. Research has determined that merely the taste of sweetness, whether by sugar or a sugar substitute, is enough to change brain chemistry in a way that mimics illegal addictive drugs such as morphine and heroin. It increases the activity of neurotransmitters known as *beta-endorphins,* which suppress the sensation of pain, boost feelings of well-being, and promote relaxation. Like the repercussions of regular sugar intake, once you build a tolerance to artificial sweeteners, it becomes difficult to function properly without them in your diet. It not only triggers cravings for unhealthful foods but also makes unsweetened, healthful whole foods taste bland and unappealing. Unfortunately, it seems as though sweeteners of any kind create a very dangerous equation that often equals addiction and disease.

TESTIMONIALS

Mike Adams and I aren't the only ones who are spreading the word about soda addiction. Certified eating disorder specialist and best-selling author Kay Sheppard has helped many people through the withdrawal and healing phases of food addictions.[6] As part of her research on soda addiction, Kay sent a fourteen-question survey to a group of confirmed and suspected soda addicts. The questions included:

- Are you or have you been addicted to soft drinks, sport drinks, or energy drinks?

- What was the name of the drink?

- How long have you been addicted or how long were you addicted?

- If you have stopped, how did you stop? If you are still addicted, can you talk about it?

- How has it affected your life and the lives of your family members?

- Can you recommend anything to others to help them stop drinking soda?

- Did the amount of soda you drank increase over time in order to get the desired effect?

- What withdrawal symptoms do you experience when you stop drinking soda?

- Do you ever drink soda to avoid withdrawal symptoms?

- Do you drink larger or more frequent amounts of soda than you planned?

- Have your attempts to control or cut down your use of soda been unsuccessful?

- Do you spend a great deal of time in activities necessary to obtain soda, use soda, or recover from its effects?

- Has your use of soda ever affected social, occupational, or recreational activities?

- Have you continued to use soda despite the knowledge of having persistent physical or psychological problems that are likely to have been caused or made worse by your use of soda?

While most respondents of the questionnaire did not answer every question, a number of them had very vivid stories to tell. What follows are a few of these stories. I have changed the names, but the facts are straight from the survey. If I had wanted to write fictional accounts of soda addiction, I could not have thought up better ones than the real tales you are about to read.

Lisa

For twenty-seven years, from age sixteen to age forty-three, Lisa drank the diet cola Tab. She started with two cans per day, and by the end of her addiction she was drinking as many as six. She could never get enough. Her doctor told her that diet soft drinks leach calcium out of bone, and that Lisa would end up with osteoporosis by age fifty if her habit persisted. Lisa stopped cold turkey and asked God to help her persevere through the discomfort of withdrawal. Without soda she experienced a drop in blood sugar and felt a lack of motivation. She wanted to isolate herself and not be around anyone. Mental fogginess, shakiness, irritability, lack of energy, sleepiness, and moodiness were all part of her daily emotional states. She constantly thought of having just a little sip of

Soft Drinks and
General Adaptation Syndrome

There is often an element of bodily stress that leads to addictions such as those that you will read about on the following pages. According to Dr. Hans Selye's book *The Stress of Life*,[5] stressors cause the body to go through three reactionary phases, which together make up a process called *General Adaptation Syndrome* (GAS). The three stages are alarm, resistance, and exhaustion. Although this concept was first applied to psychological stress, it has since been broadened to include any type of stress encountered by the body, including food allergies, of which soft drinks are a good example. In light of this fact, I find it easier to understand the phases of GAS through the use of the following terms: allergy and addiction, adaptation, and degeneration.

When you consume large amounts of a food or drink over and over again, it is not uncommon to become allergic to it, particularly if it is already harmful to your system. The human body was not meant to handle large amounts of abusive foods on a regular basis. Doing so causes the body to lose its ability to maintain homeostasis. Soft drinks contain many substances that can promote an allergic reaction, including sugar, sugar substitutes, and caffeine. Sometimes a reaction is the result of a combination of ingredients. Often it can occur as a *masked allergy*, meaning that the allergen affects your system without you even realizing it. (This is especially scary because it means that you don't realize what the soft drink is doing to you until your body enters phase

Tab to ease the withdrawal symptoms, not understanding the craziness of that idea.

Thankfully, Lisa's cravings eventually subsided and her knowledge of the danger of soft drinks eliminated any desire to pick up the habit again. She did, however, develop osteoporosis at age fifty-two. The addiction took its toll not only on Lisa but also on her family. They had to pay the medical cost of osteoporosis treatment and were continually concerned about Lisa's level of activity, always worried she might break a bone.

three and becomes exhausted.) To deal with the stress, your body releases chemicals such as adrenaline, marking phase one of GAS. It is during this phase that you can become addicted to the drink. You begin wanting more of it because it actually makes you feel great. The problem is that this feeling lasts for only a short period of time. Once that time has passed, you start to feel unwell, experiencing symptoms of withdrawal that may include headaches, fatigue, anger, and depression. (Both allergy and addiction can cause feelings of withdrawal, which each person can experience differently.) This starts a vicious cycle of drinking, feeling well for a short period, experiencing symptoms of withdrawal, and then drinking again.

If you continue to consume soft drinks, your body will enter phase two, resistance. In this phase, your body begins to adapt itself to tolerate chronic stress and cope with the allergen. At this point, other symptoms that lead to degenerative disease can occur, including joint pain, swelling of the hands and feet, yeast infections, allergies to different foods, and chronic fatigue, to mention a few. By continuing to drink soda and keeping your system in an almost constant state of stress, your body will eventually enter stage three, exhaustion. At this point, your system begins to break down, allowing illness and disease to take root.

Luckily, you can take steps to reverse this syndrome. The medical profession may not yet recognize the importance of GAS in relation to the proliferation of disease in this country, but soda drinkers should take note. You can stop this tragic cycle of events before it ends in disaster and heal yourself.

Joan

Joan started drinking Pepsi as a substitute for smoking cigarettes, which she had recently quit. She increased her intake continually to help her feel better. After a year, she realized that she had become addicted to the drink and had to remove it from her life as she had cigarettes. She tried to cut down, but was unsuccessful. She began to drink orange soda instead of cola, allowing herself to believe that its lack of caffeine somehow made it okay. (It's amazing the lengths someone can go to in denial of an addiction.) Eventually she decided that she might as well get it over with and quit cold turkey, just as she had done with nicotine.

Her withdrawal symptoms included headaches and frequent irritability. Joan was so often grumpy at work that her boss practically demanded that she have a Pepsi to improve her mood. Although the symptoms eventually stopped, Pepsi addiction had already left its mark on Joan. From drinking all of that soda, she had gained far too much weight and was now self-conscious about her appearance.

Louise

Even in her earliest memories, soft drinks were the only beverage Louise ever wanted. As a child, she actually looked down on anyone who offered her water, which she assumed was for second-class citizens! Louise always had a soda in her hand, but she wasn't loyal to any particular brand. For years she was addicted to all sorts of soft drinks. She started with Coke, moved on to Diet Rite, and later switched to caffeine-free Dr Pepper. She drank soda everywhere she went and became grumpy if she had to go without one. Although soft drinks never seemed to quench her thirst, she kept drinking them, one after another.

She had constant cravings and always needed a cold can of soda. She found herself going to the fridge without even thinking about it. She would stand at the open door for a few minutes before she realized that she was there to get a soft drink. Despite not allowing her children to drink it, despite knowing it was bad for her health, despite not wanting to want it, soda still dominated Louise diet. It is truly amazing how hard it is to give up soft drinks!

Louise quit the habit, but not cold turkey. She did it gradually by switching over to decaffeinated sweet tea and slowly making the tea less and less sweet. She cut the sugar in her tea down to nothing and began to drink unsweetened decaffeinated tea. Eventually she switched to plain water.

Sue

Sue, a recovering alcoholic, became addicted to Coke at age fourteen. At age twenty-two, she became concerned about the calories in Coke and switched to Diet Coke. (Little did she know that calories and weight would be the least of her concerns.) Although Diet Coke was not as satisfying in the beginning, she knew it was an acquired taste, so she forced herself to like it. This addiction lasted until she was twenty-seven years old, at which point she switched drinks again, this time to Coke Zero.

Sue was immediately hooked. It was an entirely different soft drink experience for her. She had Coke Zero blackouts similar to those she had known as an alcoholic. She discovered that this strange side effect was most likely the result of an allergy to the acesulfame potassium (ace K) sweetener in Coke Zero. She tried to switch back to Diet Coke but was unsuccessful. It didn't give her the same fix as Coke Zero. The addiction was so intense and progressive that in the course of one year, this 120-pound woman went from drinking twenty ounces of Coke Zero every day to consuming eight liters (that's about 270 ounces!) a day. She was not able to drive more than twenty miles without stopping to get a Coke Zero. If she couldn't find it at the store, she became extremely anxious and could not focus on anything else until she found a place that had Coke Zero in stock. She was so embarrassed by the habit that she devised a method of concealing bottles in her purse so that it looked as though she was drinking just one bottle throughout the day.

Toward the end of her Coke Zero addiction, she could not leave her house. She went from her bed to the refrigerator to bathroom, and that was all. Coke Zero had taken over her entire life. Already familiar with substance abuse, she knew what she had to do. She entered rehab.

The withdrawal symptoms from Coke Zero—anxiety, shakes, and tremors—were practically identical to those she had encountered when she quit alcohol. According to Sue, her experience with Coke Zero was in a league of its own. Diet Coke and Coca-

Cola did not have the same effect on her brain. No other substance had ever provoked the reaction that ace k had created in her body. And although she no longer touches Coke Zero, she still dreams about it.

Joe

For over forty years, Joe, a diabetic, was addicted to all sorts of sugar-free soda. He started with Tab at the age of twenty and finally quit all soft drinks by the time he reached the age of sixty-two. Although he drinks only water now, he was never without a can, bottle, or cup of soda while he was addicted. He guarded his stash of soft drinks and would get angry when his supply ran out. He even avoided restaurants that did not carry his favorite brands. Although his diabetes got worse over the years, Joe's thirst for soda seemed unquenchable. When he eventually quit, he did so cold turkey, and recommends this method to other addicts.

CONCLUSION

If you can relate to any aspect of the previous stories, you too may be a soda addict. If you find yourself unable to function properly without these products in your diet, or your soft drink consumption has increased over time, or you joke about being "addicted" to a particular soda, you may actually be living with a problem that isn't a joke. You may truly have an addiction. The examples outlined above show just how habit-forming soda can be. In many cases, a soft drink habit is just as bad as a tobacco or alcohol addiction. And while some people can quit soda cold turkey, others must use a more gradual approach, weaning themselves off the drink by degrees. How you quit is less important than actually quitting. Whichever method works for you is the right one.

7

Marketing Madness

Defensive tackle Mean Joe Greene has had a tough day on the field dealing with an offensive line that had his number. He walks down the stadium tunnel with his jersey thrown over his shoulder. It seems long and bleak. A young fan stops him and offers up a Coke and a smile. Mean Joe drains the bottle, thanks the boy, and tosses him his jersey as thanks for brightening up his day.

If you watched television in 1980, chances are you saw that advertisement. It was so popular that it won a Clio Award for outstanding commercial and has been adapted, parodied, and imitated countless times over the years. But was it essential to the sales of Coca-Cola?

THE POWER OF ADVERTISING

From all the information you read in the previous chapter, you now know that soft drinks and other sweetened beverages can be utterly addictive. They are so clearly habit-forming that you might think soft drink producers could simply stock store shelves with their products and watch the money roll in without spending a dime on advertising. You would be wrong. The following are a few of the very successful ad campaigns put forth by soft drink companies.

Coca-Cola

The Mean Joe Greene ad illustrates exactly the despicable goal of soft drink advertisers, which is to create an emotional connection to a product that is essentially sugar water. What is worse in this case is that it targets the young. A friendly football star accepting a gift from a young boy produces warm and fuzzy feelings in boys of that age group. They will think it is cool to drink Coke because Mean Joe drinks it. Associations such as these can set up a life-long habit of unhealthful soda consumption without kids even realizing it.

The ad actually contains numerous untruths. One prime example is the bottle featured in the television spot. At the time the commercial was made, no sports stadium offered soda in glass bottles. Litter and safety concerns had long since banished glass from arenas altogether. But Coke had trademarked the "contour bottle" design, and because several decades of market research said that customers responded to it, the classic glass bottle was used in the ad. After all the hard work put into marketing by the Coca-Cola Company, is it any wonder that teenage boys drink more soda than any other demographic group? Sadly, they were specifically targeted.

Diet Pepsi

Pepsi capitalized on the success of the movie *Top Gun* in the 1980s with a Diet Pepsi commercial that featured two Navy jets flying in formation. In the ad, one pilot can't get his bottle of Diet Pepsi out of the storage space near his seat. The other pilot teases him, which provokes the first pilot to roll his plane over into an inverted position so that gravity can drain the bottle into his cup. Interestingly, a member of my research staff happened to witness a group of college students as they watched this commercial from a lounge in their dorm. Immediately after seeing it, one of the students got up, marched into the elevator, and took it down to the lobby where he bought a Diet Pepsi.

Gatorade

In an ad campaign for Gatorade, athletes are shown sweating profusely as they play their chosen sport. The entire content of the commercial is shown in black and white, except for the sweat drops, which have been colored to match particular flavors of Gatorade. By the end of the spot, the viewer is asked a question by Gatorade's slogan: "Is it in you?" Clearly, the company is linking Gatorade to sweat, suggesting that the elements lost through perspiration can only be properly restored in the body by drinking their product, which, in reality, is mostly sugar and water. I don't know about you, but my sweat has always come out clear.

By combining the previously mentioned ad campaign with their other commercials, some of which star sports heroes Lebron James and Eli Manning, Gatorade has created a powerful association between their unhealthful drinks and the popular pastime of sports. You may even consider Gatorade a necessary part of playing sports, which could not be further from the truth.

Vitamin Water

Some drink manufacturers could be accused of outright lying in their advertisements. The Coca-Cola Company, the parent corporation of Vitamin Water, was, in fact, criticized for advertising the product as a "healthful alternative" to soda and sued by the Center for Science in the Public Interest for "deliberately deceiving" consumers through marketing. With an average of 33 grams of sugar per bottle, Vitamin Water does more to promote obesity and disease than it does to achieve the touted health benefits of its vitamin and mineral content.

As you learned in Chapter 4, Vitamin Water names its flavors after snappy and empowering buzzwords such as "defense," "energy," "essential," "focus," and "revive." But do you really think you're restoring balance to your body by ingesting 33 grams of sugar? Do you think this fortified sugar water is really going to promote endurance? At this point in the book, I'm sure you know better, but don't tell that to Coke's former chairman and CEO M. Douglas Ivester, who made the following statement while defending the company's marketing practices in Africa: "Actually, our product is quite healthy. Fluid replenishment is a key to health. Coca-Cola does a great service because it encourages people to take in more and more liquids." When did the Brooklyn Bridge come up for sale?

THE POWER OF PROMOTIONAL MATERIALS

Of the billions of marketing dollars spent annually by soft drink corporations such as Coca-Cola and Pepsi, a portion is always put towards the creation of promotional materials. These days, a wide variety of items are stamped with corporate logos for advertising purposes. Key chains, bottle openers, t-shirts, and baseball caps are among the most popular giveaways used by soda manufacturers to keep your mind on their product.

Another sought-after promotional tool is the movie tie-in. When a company acquires marketing rights to a film, those rights could translate into substantial profit, particularly if the film turns out to be successful. A perfect example of the power of the movie tie-in occurred in 2001, when Coca-Cola paid $150 million to Warner Brothers for the marketing rights to *Harry Potter and the Sorcerer's Stone*, expertly riding the Harry Potter wave. Limited edition bottles and cans promoting the film were created, and pictures of Harry Potter and other characters from the movie could be found wherever Coke products were sold. The series went on to make billions at the box office, and Coca-Cola was able to reap a significant reward for its continued association with the blockbuster flicks. Moreover, the partnership allowed Coca-Cola to reach the impressionable youth market, possibly fostering loyal lifetime customers.

GIVE THEM MORE OF WHAT THEY WANT

Clever advertisements and promotions are undoubtedly effective ways to get you hooked on a certain type of soft drink. But I think

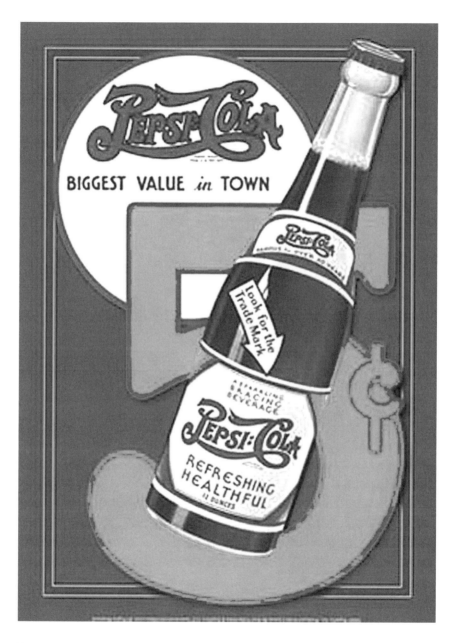

This vintage ad promotes Pepsi's twelve-ounce bottle, which seems small by today's standards. Note how the label markets the drink as "healthful," a term that couldn't be further from the truth.

it is fair to say that these tools have been helped by the ever-increasing size of soft drink containers over the years. If soda is addictive because of its bubbly water and sweet flavor, why not give customers more of what they crave, right?

In 1951, Coca-Cola came in a six-ounce bottle. These days, the smallest containers of Coke are twelve-ounce cans and twenty-ounce bottles. The problem is that these sizes do not reflect just one serving. The twenty-ounce bottle actually contains two and half servings of soda. Because soft drinks lose their carbonation once opened and flat soda is unappealing, most people down a whole container in one sitting. That means you're almost guaranteed to drink two and a half times the calories, sweetener, and other ingredients listed on the label without even realizing how much you've consumed.

LIGHTS, CAMERA, COLA!

Television commercials and movie tie-ins aren't the only means by which soft drink manufacturers attempt to reach potential consumers. Over the years, soda companies have discovered that *product placement*—the appearance of a particular brand of product within a television show or movie—can be an extremely useful marketing method. (This fact is especially true now that technology has made it so easy for television viewers to fast-forward through commercials.) Instead of using a fictional brand, filmmakers receive money from a company to feature its product on-screen. Whether it is the use of Coca-Cola in *The Gods Must Be Crazy* or Pepsi in *Back to the Future,* by having their product incorporated into the story of a film or television program, soft drink companies can rest assured that it will be seen.

When a placement is done well, the product's appearance is subtle and covert, allowing the advertisement to be absorbed unknowingly by the viewer, and sometimes even lending the product credibility through its association with a popular television or movie star. Unfortunately, a Michigan State media survey showed that the younger the audience for a television show, the more likely the story would depict the consumption of junk food, such as soda, without displaying any of the typical consequences of that consumption.[1]

LOCATION, LOCATION, LOCATION

The most obvious way that soda companies stay successful is availability. From train stations to college campuses, soft drink vending machines are practically everywhere. I walk past them every time I take my car in to be serviced. They are almost impossible to avoid. Perhaps the most coveted place to have a vending machine is anywhere groups of children gather. As previously mentioned, getting kids hooked early is an important part of establishing brand loyalty. In fact, Coca-Cola paid $60 million over ten years for the exclusive right to sell their products in the various chapters of The Boys and Girls Clubs of America.

Although all soda companies know the monetary value of having their drinks in schools, recently, a serious debate erupted over soft drink vending machines remaining at these locations. Some school systems continue to allow them, and others have had them removed. While schools that have the machines are able to increase their revenues by collecting marketing fees from the soda companies, studies have shown that children of schools that have eliminated the machines tend to score better on tests.

Another cute marketing trick can be seen in supermarkets and corner stores across the country. It is simply the act of placing soft drinks next to the foods that are typically associated with them, such as potato chips, pretzels, and dips. Research shows that sales of both soda and chips increase by 9 percent when the two products appear in the same supermarket aisle, but decrease when they are separated by at least one aisle.

STRANGE BEDFELLOWS

You should be able to trust what your family physician tells you about soft drinks, right? While your doctor might not be aware of *every* dangerous effect that sugar, high-fructose corn syrup, and the chemicals found in soda can have on your body, the information you *do* receive should be objective and unbiased, right? There shouldn't be any reason to suspect that the advice of your family physician might be tainted by a conflict of interest between his professional organization and a major soda company, should there? Perhaps you should think again.

In 2009, the American Academy of Family Physicians (AAFP) signed a marketing agreement with Coca-Cola for $500,000. The partnership was created to educate consumers on the subject of sugary beverages such as soda so that they might make informed decisions while trying to maintain a healthful lifestyle. It appeared as though Coca-Cola was up to its usual tricks, paying off potential adversaries to downplay any new information that might hurt its sales. Understandably, critics of the partnership felt that doctors might be encouraged to soft-pedal the strong connection between soft drinks and health problems such as obesity, or promote the consumption of diet drinks, which might be just as bad for you.[2] My position is that there is no way to incorporate soft drinks of any kind into a healthful diet. Just take another look at Chapter 5 to see all the diseases and health conditions that have been linked to soda. It's true that cutting down on soft drink consumption will be somewhat helpful, but stopping completely has to be the ultimate goal.

A POISON BY ANY OTHER NAME

Another thing to watch out for is when a beverage or an ingredient of a beverage decides to re-brand itself under another name. A truly despicable example of this practice recently occurred when the world's leading supplier of the artificial sweetener aspartame, which is generally sold under the name NutraSweet, decided to market the additive under the name AminoSweet. In light of the decades of increasingly bad press that aspartame has received since being introduced in 1965—the worst of which linked the sweetener to brain tumors and other types of cancer—

I'm sure it seemed like the perfect time to give the chemical a new name. So, in hopes of extending sales of aspartame and latching on to the current trend towards natural sweeteners, AminoSweet was born.

The name, which references the fact that aspartame is made of two amino acids, is an attempt to paint the sweetener as simply a combination of naturally occurring substances. But, in reality, the combination of aspartic acid and phenylalanine does not occur anywhere in nature. The truth is that aspartame is about as artificial as it gets, no matter what you call it.

The whole situation reminds me of the many different names adopted by the intelligence service and secret police of the Soviet Union before 1954, when they were finally reorganized as the KGB. Whatever it was called, the KGB was still the same brutal security agency that performed legal and illegal espionage to protect the state. The truth is that corporations will do anything to sell you a product, including changing its name to make it seem like something different, which is essentially a legal form of lying. Don't be fooled.[3]

CONCLUSION

Once you take the time to think about it, the amount of marketing to which you are exposed on a daily basis is frightening. Advertisements are everywhere, whether they appear on billboards, in the form of television commercials, or on t-shirts that are given away at sporting events. Additionally, when beverage companies such as Coca-Cola and Pepsi aren't trying to promote their products directly, they are doing their best to reach your subconscious mind, paying large amounts of money to have their drinks incorporated into movies and television programs.

It is one thing when these strategies are aimed at adults—we should know better—but it is quite another when they target children. And while parents can exert a certain amount of control over what their kids see, their job is made almost impossible when vending machines full of soda are virtually everywhere, including schools and after-school clubs. It is no wonder that the soda habit is so easily picked up and so extremely difficult to give up. But now that you have a good idea of the forces at work against you, it is time you learned what you can do to beat them and end your addiction.

8

How to
Solve the Problem

You now know how important homeostasis, or balance, is to your body. You also know about the unhealthful ingredients found in soft drinks and other sweetened beverages, and the way in which they can knock your body out of balance. But, as explained in Chapter 7, these drinks can be addictive, and beverage manufacturers are constantly trying to tempt you into buying their habit-forming products. Advertisements for soft drinks are everywhere you look. With the odds of avoiding or kicking the habit so stacked against you, it's legitimate to wonder if you even stand a chance.

The truth is that there are techniques you can use to beat these challenges. In addition, your chance at success is strengthened when your community and government get involved. This chapter details common-sense steps that you and the people around you can take to change your health, your family's health, and the health of this country for the better. This pressing problem can be solved if we each do our part.

WHAT YOU CAN DO

The first step on the road to wellness is a personal one. In order to conquer an addiction to soda or any other sweetened drink, you must first learn what you can do for yourself. The following are tips to help you achieve your goal.

- Instead of going cold turkey, make the change a little at a time. Cut back on your soda consumption slowly. If, for instance, you drink two cans a day, start by cutting back to one can a day. Continue to gradually eliminate your consumption. Most people find it much easier to stop this way.

- Substitute water for soft drinks. Take the money you would normally spend on soft drinks and put it into a jar each day. At the end of the month, buy yourself a gift with the money you've saved.

- If switching to plain water is too difficult initially, find a different substitute. (See the inset "Soft Drink Substitutes" on page 90.) Make sure you have one of these alternatives in your home at all times.

- Don't buy soft drinks when you go grocery shopping. If that's too hard, send someone else to do your shopping for you. If you don't have soda in your home, there is less of a chance that you'll drink it.

- As a challenge, try to go one week without a soft drink. Give yourself a reward once you have met the challenge. Reward is a good motivator.

- Let your friends and family know that you are giving up soft drinks. It is harder to go back on your commitment once others know about it.

- Regularly read about the negative effects that soft drinks can have on your health. (See Chapter 5.) That may be enough to scare you into avoiding them.

- Recognize that soft drink addiction can be as serious as any other addiction and treat it accordingly. Just as an alcoholic cannot have even a sip of liquor, indulging in a little taste of soda every now and again can be a problem for most soda addicts.

- Ask a friend or family member to be your "sponsor." Commonly used by members of Alcoholics Anonymous and other twelve-step programs, a sponsor is someone you can call to help you deal with your cravings, which can be too difficult to deal with on your own at times. Support is the key to success.

- In much the same way that Alcoholics Anonymous helps alcoholics conquer their addiction, there are twelve-step organizations designed to help you kick your soda habit. Food Addicts Anonymous and Food Addicts in Recovery Anonymous offer meetings in communities throughout the country and are each doing an excellent job helping food and drink addicts end their substance abuse. Recovery from Food Addiction is a group of therapists that deal with food addiction, working with both individuals and groups. (For contact information, see the Resources on page 103.)

- There are also online resources that can help you rid yourself of sugar addiction. Author Connie Bennett has an excellent website called Stop Sugar Shock! This site offers seminars and other information on how to beat sugar addiction, which is often the basis of soda addiction. (For contact information, see the Resources on page 103.)

Perhaps the most important tip, however, is simply to make up your mind to quit. There cannot be any ifs, ands, or buts about it. If you don't want to quit soda wholeheartedly, you won't follow through with any of the previous advice. But when you truly decide to do something, you set an idea in motion that is very hard to stop.

WHAT YOUR COMMUNITY CAN DO

Although the first step in this process belongs to you alone, the second step can be aided considerably by a supportive community. Physicians, nurses, dietitians, and nutritionists should make a point to ask their patients how much soda they drink on a daily

Soft Drink Substitutes

When you've been drinking soft drinks for so long, switching to plain water can be quite a shock. If you are finding it hard to make such a big transition, perhaps a different soda substitute might help you along the road to recovery from soft drink addiction. But it can be difficult to find a suitable replacement when so many of the options contain tons of sugar. A healthy body can metabolize eight grams, or a little over two teaspoons, of sugar at one sitting. That is the criterion I used when choosing the following beverages. I sincerely hope that more choices come on the market as people begin to understand what soft drinks are doing to their health.

While some flavored waters include more sugar than I recommend, a few do not contain any sugar or calories. Brands like Metromint and Hint offer purified water that has been lightly flavored with natural essences. Metromint, as the name suggests, focuses on mint-based tastes, with varieties such as Peppermint, Lemonmint, and Choco-latemint. Hint offers fruity flavors, including Raspberry-Lime, Water-melon, and Pear.

Although coconut water contains natural sugars, I still recommend it as a possible soda substitute. Nature Factor Organic Coconut Water sells its product unflavored, while Zico mixes its coconut water with natural flavors to create drinks such as Zico Lima Citron, Zico Mango, and Zico Passion Fruit. Because the sugar content is more the eight grams per container size, I must suggest that you drink only an amount

basis. These healthcare providers should also suggest dietary adjustments to patients when appropriate. In addition, organizations that deal with women's health, children's health, dental and bone health, and heart health should collaborate on campaigns to reduce soft drink consumption. They should also push soft drink companies not to advertise to children and adolescents. Thankfully, some food companies have already promised not to advertise their products on television to children twelve and under. I think this is a move in the right direction.

that offers no more than my recommended sugar limit at one time. In other words, if a fourteen-ounce bottle includes twelve grams of sugar, do your best to drink about half the bottle, saving half for later. As an added bonus, you'll protect not only your health but also your wallet!

Sometimes it's not just the flavoring that you miss from soft drinks, it's also the carbonation. As you know, just as the sweeteners in beverages are bad for your health, the carbon dioxide in fizzy drinks produces negative effects in your system, too. For that reason, I don't like to recommend bubbly drinks outright. I understand, however, that they can be helpful in weaning you off soda. If you must have a fizzy drink, try R.W. Knudsen Family's Sparkling Essence beverages. They feature natural flavors such as lemon extract and blueberry extract, and are free of any sweeteners. Additionally, you could simply mix your own choice of pure fruit juice with carbonated water to create a personalized concoction. Just be sure that the serving of juice does not exceed eight grams of sugar.

Finally, for those of you who have a little more time on your hands and want to keep costs down, caffeine-free tea might be your answer. Place two tea bags in a container, add a quart of boiling water, and let the tea steep for at least thirty minutes. Remove the tea bags and refrigerate for refreshing iced tea. (The tea should keep about a week in the refrigerator.) My favorite flavors are Good Earth brand's Sweet and Spicy Tea (both original and organic), as well as Bigelow's Red Raspberry Herbal Tea. Thankfully, each of the soft drink substitutes mentioned in this section can be purchased at most independent and chain retailers.

Another positive step came with the recent establishment of the School Beverage Guidelines, with which virtually all schools now comply. Created jointly by the Alliance for a Healthier Generation and the American Beverage Association, these strong and important guidelines call for the removal of all sugar-sweetened soft drinks from schools, including kindergarten through twelfth grade. High schools, however, are still allowed no-calorie and low-calorie drinks that contain no more than sixty calories per eight-ounce serving.[1]

Unfortunately, young children attend birthday parties and other celebrations that may include soda. And soft drinks continue to be given out liberally after kids' athletic events, when a bottle of water and an orange would actually do better to quench a child's thirst. While I do understand that they need the money, youth organizations should not auction themselves off to the highest bidder for sponsorship by a soft drink corporation or any other junk food company. Those deals benefit the organizations and corporations but never the children's health.

WHAT YOUR GOVERNMENT CAN DO

Would you believe that you can still buy soft drinks with government food stamps? You can also use them to buy candy, potato chips, and chewing gum. According to the Department of Agriculture, sugary drinks account for approximately 6 percent of purchases made with food stamps throughout the country. This statistic means that in New York City, where 1.7 million people receive food stamps, the government essentially subsidizes $75 million worth of sugary drinks per year. This is a great example of a much-needed adjustment in government policy. While the ultimate decision to end your soda addiction and change your life can be made only by you, your government can lend a helping hand by crafting laws that not only encourage healthful habits but also discourage unhealthful ones.

A good way to start the process would be to end sugar and corn subsidies. By subsidizing these commodities, the government is making sweeteners such as sucrose and high-fructose corn syrup cheap, and thus promoting the creation and consumption of inexpensive sugary foods, including soda. Why buy fruits and vegetables when it is cheaper to fill up on a bottle of Dr Pepper, right? Unfortunately, sugar and corn growers are well organized. They protect their subsidies by providing large campaign donations to the politicians who support them. This must change. We would all be better off if the government subsidized healthful fruits and vegetables instead.

As mentioned in Chapter 7, soft drink vending machines are practically everywhere. If you are a soda addict, the outside world is a tough place to navigate without giving in to your habit. One solution that local, state, and federal governments could try would be to place more water fountains in public buildings and other spaces. It is such a simple idea that could be so powerful. Wherever a vending machine is found, a water fountain should be close by. At least give us a fighting chance to make the right choice.

Perhaps the most powerful way in which governments can help solve the problem of soft drink addiction is through taxation. In a Harvard University study, researchers manipulated the price of soft drinks at two hospital cafeterias in Boston to determine its effect on soda consumption. They found that when the cost of soda increased by 35 percent, sales declined by 26 percent at both hospitals. When the researchers simply provided education on the adverse health effects of soda but did not increase cost, consumption did not decline at all. Finally, when education was provided *and* the price of soda was raised, results showed a 44-percent decrease in the sale of soft drinks.[2]

While a few states have, in fact, added a very small tax on soft drinks, the revenue from that tax is generally not used to support physical education in schools, build swimming pools and bike paths, or create campaigns that promote a healthful diet. A soft drink tax should be used not only as a means of reducing soda consumption (and thereby lowering healthcare costs) but also as a way to generate revenue that governments can put towards health programs.

A poll of New York State residents showed that 52 percent of respondents would support a soda tax. In addition, 72 percent would support such a tax if the revenue were used to fund programs dedicated to the prevention of obesity. It seems as though the way in which the issue is framed is important to its acceptance. Support for the tax is highest when it is introduced to encourage health and when the revenue is earmarked for programs that promote childhood nutrition or obesity prevention.[3] In light of the above-mentioned study and poll, implementing a tax on soda would be a great benefit to society.

Some local governments are doing the right thing. Official San Francisco city policy now bars vending machines from selling sugary drinks—including regular soft drinks, sports drinks, energy drinks, and enhanced waters—on public property. Juice must be 100-percent fruit or vegetable juice with no added sweeteners, and diet soda can account for no more than 25 percent of the items offered. Following this positive trend, other cities such as San Antonio and Boston have also begun to restrict sugary drinks in one fashion or another.

History shows us that governmental intervention can spark positive changes in society. After California banned the sale of soft drinks in elementary and middle schools in 2003, a number of other states took similar action. The legislation's ripple effect was also evident in 2006, when the American Beverage Association (comprised of the leading soft drink manufacturers) voluntarily teamed with health advocacy group the Alliance for a Healthier Generation to create the School Beverage Guidelines, which, as previously mentioned, removed all sugar-sweetened soft drinks from schools, including kindergarten through twelfth grade.

In addition to protecting the health of children by keeping soft drinks out of their hands, governments have taken steps to educate adults about the dangers of drinking soda. In 2009, the New York City Department of Health launched a massive advertising campaign called "Pouring on the Pounds" to warn people of the health consequences of soda consumption. On a national level, the FDA recently proposed a rule that would require restaurants and other types of eateries to post calorie counts on their menus. Designed to sensitize consumers to the nutritional cost of high-calorie foods, among which soft drinks are a major player, this policy is an idea that I've long supported. Information can be a powerful ally. And even if we already know the facts, it's always good to be reminded of them at an appropriate time, such as the moment you order a meal.

CONCLUSION

Like any chemical dependence, soda addiction is a very tough opponent to beat. By following a few of the tips mentioned in this chapter, you can successfully end your obsession with soft drinks and transition to a healthy life free of unhealthful sweeteners and harmful chemical additives. Although most of the responsibility lies on your shoulders, the support of your community and government can really make the difference between kicking your soda habit and falling back into the old routine. While each of these bodies has made strides towards the encouragement of healthier living, there is much more that could and should be done. So try to make changes in your community and become active in the political process. There is no time to waste. By thinking of the big picture, you will not only help others but also yourself.

Conclusion

I have said many times that knowledge is power. It is the most important factor when it comes to maintaining your health and promoting the well-being of society in general. You need to understand that soda and other sweetened drinks can be highly addictive and are filled with substances that often result in health problems over time. As you now know, balance is necessary for a healthy body. Soda and other sugary drinks lead to imbalance, and it is this imbalance that can lead to disease. The problem really is that simple to articulate, if not solve. As there are many outside forces working against you, I only hope the information on soda marketing (see Chapter 7) has helped you realize the many ways in which corporations try to manipulate you, spending billions to convince you to buy products that will most likely cause your painful demise. I just can't say it enough: Knowledge is power. Ultimately, I wrote *Killer Colas* to empower you.

Hopefully, if you are a soft drink addict, you now have enough knowledge to end your habit. Even better, if you are not yet an addict, you may now know enough to change your ways before you become addicted. Most importantly, your newfound knowledge must include the realization that you are not alone. For me, soft drinks were only a small part of my unhealthful sugar regimen. (I would be more likely to go nuts with chocolate.)

Nevertheless, I could not have become healthy without taking soda out of my diet. And even with the limited amount of soda I drank, cutting it out of my life was very hard. My point is that many people have faced the problem that you are facing right now, and many people have overcome it. You can beat back the cravings. You can stop the late-night trips to the refrigerator. People have conquered this difficult obsession. You can, too.

You can choose to be healthy, sidestepping unhealthy sweetened drinks, which have been linked to a variety of illnesses, including allergies and even cancer. You now know that there are ways to eliminate these sickening beverages from your life for good. You also know that when you join your effort to the efforts of your community and government, success is more than just possible, it is likely. The fact is that you are no longer the helpless victim that you were before opening this book. Now that you have read *Killer Colas,* you have knowledge and, therefore, you have power. Use it. Change your life as well as the health of this country—and maybe even the world.

Glossary

acesulfame potassium (acesulfame K, ace K). An artificial sweet-ener made from acetoacetic acid (a weak acid) and potassium.

anaphylaxis (anaphylactic shock). A severe allergic reaction to a substance in the environment that occurs almost immediately upon exposure and includes symptoms such as itchiness, palpitations, light-headedness, difficulty swallowing, and difficulty breathing. The most severe cases of anaphylaxis result in complete closure of the airways, shock, and death.

ascorbic acid. A form of vitamin C that not only restores some of the nutritional value lost during the processing of a beverage but also acts as an antioxidant that helps improve color and taste.

aspartame. An artificial sweetener that consists of methanol and the amino acids aspartic acid and phenylalanine.

bisphenol A. Chemical used in the production of polycarbonate plastics as well as epoxy resins. Most commonly found in beverage bottles, baby bottles, and the lining of aluminum cans, BPA is known to leach out of these containers, particularly when they are in contact with high-temperature or acidic liquids. When bisphenol A accumulates in the body, it can disrupt normal hormone function, resulting in health problems. Children are particularly sensitive to this chemical.

body mass index (BMI). A number used to indicate a person's level of body fat, which is calculated from an individual's height and weight.

citric acid. A naturally occurring acid found in citrus fruits and berries. It is added to fruit-flavored soft drinks to give them a tangy flavor and also acts as a preservative.

crystalline fructose. A sweetener processed from corn and composed almost entirely of fructose.

degenerative disease. A disease marked by the deterioration of a tissue, organ, or bodily function.

esophagus. An organ composed of a muscular tube lined with a mucous membrane that connects the throat to the stomach.

epilepsy. A disorder that causes repeated seizures as a result of nerve cells in the brain firing electrical impulses at a rate of up to four times higher than normal.

food additive. A synthetic or natural substance added to food to preserve flavor or enhance taste and appearance.

fructose. A simple sugar commonly found in fruits and vegetables. It is metabolized solely by the liver.

functional beverage. A drink designed for a specific purpose aside from just quenching thirst. A functional beverage usually includes non-traditional ingredients, such as herbs, vitamins, minerals, and amino acids, depending on its intended purpose. Examples of this type of product are sports drinks, energy drinks, and enhanced waters.

gestational diabetes. A condition in which women without previously diagnosed diabetes exhibit high blood glucose levels during pregnancy, which usually return to normal after giving birth.

glucose. A simple sugar found in most dietary carbohydrates that acts as the body's main source of energy.

glycemic index (GI). A numerical system that measures how quickly a food triggers a rise in blood glucose.

gout. A disease caused by high levels of uric acid that involves inflammation of the joints, especially of the hands and feet.

high-fructose corn syrup. A sweetener derived from corn that has been processed to increase its fructose content. It is used in almost all processed foods and beverages, including soft drinks, ketchup, yogurt, cookies, and salad dressing.

homeostasis. The ability of a living organism to adjust its internal environment to maintain a state of equilibrium. When this ability is continually impaired, disease can occur.

hypokalemia. A condition defined by a low level of potassium in the blood, which typically leads to muscular weakness.

inflammation. Redness, swelling, pain, and disturbed function in an area of the body.

insulin resistance. A condition in which insulin in the body stops metabolizing sugar effectively. As a result, the pancreas secretes more insulin into the bloodstream in an effort to reduce blood glucose levels. This throws the body out of homeostasis, leading to diabetes.

leptin. A hormone produced by adipose (fat) tissue that plays a central role in fat metabolism by helping to control appetite. It is also associated with blood cell development, blood vessel formation, and immune function.

maltodextrin. An easily digested carbohydrate generally made from cornstarch and used to sweeten shakes and as a food additive. It has a high glycemic index and can disrupt homeostasis.

metabolic syndrome. A collection of conditions, including obesity, high blood pressure, and insulin resistance, that signals an increased risk of more serious illnesses, such as heart disease, stroke, and diabetes.

neotame. An artificial sweetener that is chemically similar to aspartame but not a source of phenylalanine.

neurotransmitter. A chemical messenger in the body that transmits information from one cell to another.

osteoporosis. The loss of bone or skeletal tissue that produces brittleness or softness of bone.

pH. The measurement of the acidity or alkalinity of a solution.

phosphoric acid. A chemical that gives soda a tangy flavor and maintains its carbonation.

saccharin. An artificial sweetener that is much sweeter than sucrose but not metabolized by the body.

sodium benzoate. A preservative used by soft drink manufacturers to prevent the growth of organisms such as mold and bacteria in their products. When combined with ascorbic acid at high temperatures, it produces the carcinogenic compound known as benzene.

sodium citrate. A sodium salt of citric acid that is often included alongside citric acid to regulate the acidity of a soda. It also keeps any fats or fat-soluble compounds emulsified in a liquid.

stevia (steviol glycosides). A natural sugar substitute extracted from the stevia leaf that has virtually no effect on blood sugar.

sucralose. An artificial sweetener that the body does not break down and, therefore, has no calories.

sucrose. A sugar derived from sugar beets or cane and consisting of two simple sugars called glucose and fructose in equal amounts. It is also known as table sugar.

sugar alcohols. A sweetener that is made mainly from cornstarch and used with artificial sweeteners to enhance sweetness and flavor. Although its chemical structure resembles both sugar and alcohol, it is neither a sugar nor an alcohol.

Tourette syndrome. A disorder of the nervous system characterized by multiple physical (motor) tics and at least one vocal (phonic) tic, which come and go. Genetic and environmental factors play a role in its occurrence.

uric acid. The final result of the metabolism of purines, which are found in high levels in meat and meat products.

Resources

While cutting soda and other sugary beverages from your diet may be the toughest thing you'll ever do, there are a number of resources that can help you achieve your goal. The following groups and organizations, informative websites, and recommended products can help you stay on the right path.

GROUPS AND ORGANIZATIONS

Aspartame Consumer Safety Network (ACSN)
PO Box 2001
Frisco, TX 75034
Phone: 214-387-4001
Website: www.aspartamesafety.com

Established in 1987, this organization promotes awareness of the dangers of aspartame consumption. Its website presents news articles, peer-reviewed studies, and personal stories regarding the artificial sweetener and its side effects.

Center for Science in the Public Interest (CSPI)
1220 L Street NW, Suite 300
Washington, DC 20005
Phone: 202-332-9110
Website: www.cspinet.org

Since 1971, the Center for Science in the Public Interest (CSPI) has been a strong advocate for nutrition and health, food safety, alcohol policy, and sound science. CSPI's focus is to educate the public, advocate government policies that are consistent with scientific evidence on health and environmental issues, and counter industry's powerful influence on public opinion and public policies.

Food Addicts Anonymous (FAA)
529 NW Prima Vista Boulevard, # 301A
Port St. Lucie, FL 34983
Phone: 561-967-3871
Website: www.foodaddictsanonymous.org

Food Addicts Anonymous (FAA) treats food and/or beverage addictions as biochemical disorders and offers a twelve-step program to beat the illness. FAA helps members conquer their addiction through sound nutritional advice, abstinence from addictive products, and working the program's twelve steps through meetings, which are held throughout the world. Also offers online and telephone support. There are no dues or fees.

Food Addicts in Recovery Anonymous (FA)
400 W. Cummings Park, Suite 1700
Woburn, MA 01801
Phone: 781-932-6300
Website: www.foodaddicts.org

Based on the twelve steps of Alcoholics Anonymous, Food Addicts in Recovery Anonymous is an international organization that welcomes anyone who wants help defeating food and/or beverage addictions. There are no dues or fees to join, and meetings are available worldwide.

Mission Possible World Health International
9270 River Club Parkway
Duluth, GA 30097
Phone: 770-242-2599
Website: www.mpwhi.com

Founded by Dr. Betty Martini, this organization was formed as a means to spread the word about the deadly side effects of aspartame. Its website offers a wealth of information on the subject.

Recovery from Food Addiction (RFA)

PO Box 35543

Houston, TX 77235

Phone: 713-673-2848

Website: www.recoveryfromfoodaddiction.org

The focus of RFA is abstinence from sugar, flour, and wheat in all forms. RFA also relies on a twelve-step program to help its members successfully abstain from these additive foods through meetings, which are held throughout the United States. There are no dues or fees.

INFORMATIVE WEBSITES

Kay Sheppard
www.kaysheppard.com

A licensed mental health counselor and a certified eating disorders specialist, Kay Sheppard conducts workshops for food addicts worldwide. Through her Recovery Food Plan, Kay has helped people eliminate cravings for sugar, caffeine, carbohydrates, and more. In addition to providing information on the Food Plan, this website offers online meetings, workshops, and consultations.

Nancy Appleton, PhD
www.nancyappleton.com

This website, launched by health advocate Dr. Nancy Appleton, offers a wealth of information on the dangers of sugar. It includes a quiz to see if you are a sugarholic, a listing of "141 Reasons Why Sugar Is Ruining Your Health," a variety of healthy recipes, a number of recommended books and CDs by Dr. Appleton, and much, much more.

Neotame Toxicity Information Center
www.holisticmed.com/neotame

Run by the Holistic Healing Web Page, the Neotame Toxicity Information Center is an online resource designed to expose the unhealthful nature of neotame, an artificial sweetener that is chemically similar to aspartame.

Nutrition Data
www.nutritiondata.com

Since its launch in 2003, Nutrition Data has grown into one of the most authoritative and useful sources of nutritional analysis on the Internet. Its continuing goal is to provide accurate and comprehensive information on nutrition and healthy lifestyle choices.

Stop Sugar Shock!
www.sugarshock.com

Run by Connie Bennett, the author of Sugar Shock!, this website is designed to help you end your addiction to sugar. It contains links to helpful daily tips, fun and informative quizzes, as well as a program created by Connie that can teach you how to give up sugar for good.

Sucralose Toxicity Information Center
www.holisticmed.com/splenda

Run by the Holistic Healing Web Page, the Sucralose Toxicity Information Center is an online resource designed to expose the toxic nature of sucralose—an artificial sweetener sold under the brand name Splenda.

Sweet Poison
www.sweetpoison.com

This is the website of Janet Starr Hull, creator of the Aspartame Detoxification Program. When Janet was diagnosed with Grave's disease—a fatal thyroid disorder—she believed that her illness was actually caused by aspartame poisoning, which has symptoms that mimic Graves. After following the detoxification program she created, Janet restored her health within thirty days. Her website provides important information on the harmful effects of aspartame, detoxification guidelines, and much more.

The Truth About Splenda
www.truthaboutspenda.com

Provided by The Sugar Association, this website serves as a clearinghouse for information on the artificial sweetener sucralose, which is better known by its brand name—Splenda. It raises issues about the safety of Splenda and offers ways to take action to bring the facts about the sweetener to light.

RECOMMENDED BEVERAGE MANUFACTURERS

Bigelow Tea

R.C. Bigelow, Inc.

201 Black Rock Turnpike

Fairfield, CT 06825

Phone: 888-244-3569

www.bigelowtea.com

Bigelow produces a variety of high-quality black, green, and herbal teas. They are available at most grocery stores.

Edward & Sons Trading Company, Inc.

PO Box 1326

Carpinteria, CA 93014

Phone: 805-684-8500

Website: www.edwardandsons.com

This company offers Nature Factor Organic Coconut Water—the world's first certified organic coconut water.

Good Earth Teas

890 Mountain Avenue, Suite 105

New Providence, NJ 07974

Phone: 888-625-8227

Website: www.goodearth.com

Good Earth is one of the first American herbal companies and a leader in specialty teas. It offers many different tea blends with a variety of healthful ingredients, including ginger root, papaya, and lemongrass.

Hint, Inc.

Phone: 866-895-HINT (4468)

Website: www.drinkhint.com

This company's logo includes the phrase "Drink water, not sugar." Hint beverages are lightly flavored purified waters. They are unsweetened, pre-servative- and calorie-free, and come in a variety of flavors.

Soma Beverage Company, LLC
PO Box 885462
San Francisco, CA 94188
Phone: 415-979-0781
Website: www.metromint.com

This company produces Metromint—purified bottled water in a variety of flavors, all of which feature the essence of mint. Their products are unsweetened, free of artificial ingredients, and contain only natural flavorings.

R.W. Knudsen Family
1 Strawberry Lane
Orrville, Ohio 44667
Phone: 888-569-6993
Website: www.rwknudsenfamily.com

This company's line of flavored carbonated water drinks is called Sparkling Essence. Containing only sparkling spring water and the essence of such ingredients as lemon, mint, and cucumber, these beverages are made without artificial additives or added sugar.

Zico
643 Cypress Avenue
Hermosa Beach, CA 90254
Phone: 866-SAY-ZICO (729-9426)
Website: www.zico.com

This company's Zico Natural is 100-percent pure coconut water from young coconuts. It has no added sugar, fat, or cholesterol, and is suggested as a substitute for sports drinks due to its electrolyte content.

Recommended Reading

Absolutely Abstinent by Kay Sheppard. Palm Bay, FL: KSI, 2006.

Aspartame Disease: An Ignored Epidemic by H.J. Roberts. West Palm Beach, FL: Sunshine Sentinel Press, 2001.

Deadly Deception–Story of Aspartame by Mary Nash Stoddard. Dallas, TX: Odenwald Press, 1998.

Excitotoxins: The Taste That Kills by Russell L Blaylock, MD. Santa Fe, NM: Health Press, 2006.

Food Addiction: The Body Knows by Kay Sheppard. Deerfield Beach, FL: Health Communications, Inc, 1993.

Food Addiction: Healing Day by Day by Kay Sheppard. Deerfield Beach, FL: Health Communications, Inc, 2003.

From the First Bite by Kay Sheppard. Deerfield Beach, FL: Health Communications, Inc, 2000.

Lick the Sugar Habit by Nancy Appleton, PhD. New York: Avery, Penguin Group Inc, 1995.

Nutrition and Physical Degeneration by Weston Price, MD. La Mesa, CA: Price-Pottenger Nutrition Foundation, 2008.

Pottenger's Cats by Francis Pottenger, Jr., MD. Las Mesa, CA: Price-Pottenger Nutrition Foundation, 1995.

Suicide by Sugar by Nancy Appleton, PhD. and G.N. Jacobs. Garden City Park, NY: Square One Publishers, 2009.

Sweet Deception: Why Splenda, NutraSweet, and the FDA May Be Hazardous to Your Health by Dr. Joseph Mercola and Dr. Kendra Degen Pearsall. Nashville, TN: Nelson Books, 2006.

Sweet Poison: How the World's Most Popular Artificial Sweetener is Killing Us—My Story by Janet Starr Hull. Far Hills, NJ: New Horizons Press, 2001.

The Sweetener Trap & How to Avoid It by Beatrice Trum Hunter. Laguna Beach, CA: Basic Health Publications, 1982.

The Wisdom of the Body by Walter B. Cannon, MD, PhD. (2nd Ed.) New York: Bantam Books, 1981.

Your Body Is Your Best Doctor by Melvin Page, DDS and H. Leon Abrams, Jr. New Canaan, CT: Keats Publishing, 1972.

References

Chapter 1

1. Economic Research Service (ERS), United States Department of Agriculture (USDA). Food Availability (Per Capita) Data System. www.ers.usda.gov

Chapter 3

1. Bocarslly, M.E, et al. "High-fructose corn syrup causes characteristics of obesity in rats: increased body weight, body fat and triglyceride levels." *Pharmacol Biochem Behav* 2010; 97(1):101–106.

2. Koehler, S. and Glaros, A. "The Effect of Aspartame on Migraine Headache." *Headache: The Journal of Head and Face Pain* 2006; 28(1):10–14.

3. Ciappuccini, R, et al. "Aspartame-induced fibromyalgia, an unusual but curable cause of chronic pain." *Clin Exp Rheumatol* 2010; 28(6, suppl. 63):S131–S133.

4. Mitchell, H. *Sweeteners and Sugar Alternatives in Food Technology.* Ames, IA: Blackwell Publishing Professional, 2006.

5. "Artificial Sweeteners. Aspartame: What is the Negative Side?" www.mednet.com

6. Geuns, J.M. "Stevioside." *Phytochemistry* 2003; 34(5):913–921.

7. Chan, P.C, at al. "Toxicity and Carcinogenicity Studies of 4-Methylimidazole in F344/N Rats and B6c3f1 Mice." *Arch Toxicol* 2008; 82(1):45–53.

8. "Caramel Coloring in Soda: What You Should Know about This Innocent-Sounding Ingredient." www.huffingtonpost.com

Chapter 4

1. Heckman, M.A, et al. "Energy Drinks: An Assessment of Their Market Size, Consumer Demographics, Ingredient Profile, Functionality, and Regulations in the United States." *Comprehensive Reviews in Food Science and Food Safety* 2010; 9(3):203–307.

2. "Bottled tea beverages may contain fewer polyphenols than brewed tea." American Chemical Society (2010, August 23).
http://www.portal.acs.org/portal/asc/corg/content

Chapter 5

1. Fass, R, et al. "Predictors of heartburn during sleep in a large prospective cohort study." *Chest* 2005; 127(5):1658–1666.

2. Beyer, P, et al. "Fructose intake at current levels in the United States may cause gastrointestinal distress in normal adults." *Journ Am Diet Assoc* 2005; 105(10):1559–1566.

3. Petrus, M, et al. "Asthma and intolerance to benzoates." *Arch Pediatr* 1996; 3(10):984–987.

4. Tarlo, S.L, et al. "Asthma and anaphylactoid reactions to food additives." *Canadian Family Physician* 1993; 39:1119–1123.

5. "Sugar Intake Linked to Kids' Asthma?" www.webmd.com

6. Tarlo, S.L, et al. "Asthma and anaphylactoid reactions to food additives." *Canadian Family Physician* 1993; 39:1119–1123.

7. Warburg, O, et al. "The metabolism of tumors in the body." *J Gen Physiol* 1927; 8(6): 519–530.

8. Harry, V.N, et al. "Use of new imaging techniques to predict tumor response to therapy." *Lancet Oncol* 2010; 11(1):92–102.

9. Larsson S.C, et al. "Consumption of sugar and sugar-sweetened foods and the risk of pancreatic cancer in a prospective study." *Am J Clin Nutr* 2006; 84(5):1171–1176.

10. Chan, J.M, et al. "Sweets, sweetened beverages, and risk of pancreatic cancer in a large population-based case-control study." *Cancer Causes Control* 2009; 20(6):835–846.

11. Schernhammer, E.S, et al. "Sugar-sweetened soft drink consumption and risk of pancreatic cancer in two prospective cohorts." *Cancer Epidemiol Biomarkers Prev* 2005; 14(9):2098–2105.

12. Mueller, N.T, et al. "Soft drink and juice consumption and risk of pancreatic cancer: the Singapore Chinese Health Study." *Cancer Epidemiol Biomarkers Prev* 2010; 19(2): 447–455.

13. Hui, H, et al. "Direct spectrophotometric determination of serum fructose in pancreatic cancer patients." *Pancreas* 2009; 38(6):706–712.

14. Campbell, P.T, et al. "Dietary patterns and risk of incident gastric adenocarcinoma." *Am J Epidemiol* 2008; 167(3):295–304.

15. Lamkin, D.M, et al. "Glucose has prognostic value in ovarian cancer." *Cancer* 2009; 115(5):1021–1027.

16. Key, T.J, et al. "Carbohydrates and cancer: an overview of the epidemiological evidence." *Eur J Clin Nutr* 2007; 61(suppl. 1):S112–S121.

17. Vanderloo, M.J. "Effects of lifestyle on the onset of puberty as determinant for breast cancer." *Eur J Cancer Prev* 2007; 16(1):17–25.

18. Johnson, R.K, et al. "Dietary sugars intake and cardiovascular health: a scientific statement from the American Heart Association." *Circulation* 2009; 120(11):1101–1120.

19. Van Horn, L, et al. "Translation and Implementation of Added Sugars Consumption Recommendations: A Conference Report from the American Heart Association Added Sugars Conference 2010." *Circulation* 2010; 122(23):2470–2490.

20. "The Heart Truth drives awareness throughout American Heart Month." www.nhlbi.nih.gov

21. Lyadurai, S.J, et al. "New-onset seizures in adults: possible association with consumption of popular energy drinks." *Epilepsy* 2007; 10(3):504–508.

22. Lars, L, et al. "Consumption of Soft Drinks and Hyperactivity, Mental Distress, and Conduct Problems among Adolescents in Oslo, Norway." *Am J Public Health* 2006; 96(10):1815–1820.

23. Lipton, R.B, et al. "Aspartame as a dietary trigger of headache." *Headache* 1989; 29(2):90–92.

24. Müller-Vahl, K.R, et al. "The influence of different food and drink on tics in Tourette syndrome." *Acta Paediatr* 2008; 97(4):442–446.

25. Davis, R.E, et al. "Childhood Caffeine Tic Syndrome." *Pediatrics* 1998; 101(6):E4.

26. Nguyen, S, et al. "Sugar-sweetened beverages, serum uric acid and blood pressure in adolescents." *J Pediatr* 2009; 154(6):807–813.

27. Choi, H.K, et al. "Soft Drinks, Fructose Consumption and the Risk of Gout in Men: Prospective Cohort Study." *BMJ* 2008; 336(7639):309–312.

28. Winkelmayer, W.C, et al. "Habitual caffeine intake and the risk of hypertension in women." *JAMA* 2005; 294(18):2330–2335.

29. Ferder, L, et al. "The role of high-fructose corn syrup in metabolic syndrome and hypertension." *Curr Hypertens Rep* 2010; 12(2):105–112.

30. Tsimihoimos, V, et al. "Cola induced hypokalaemia: pathophysiological mechanisms and clinical implications." *Int J Clin Pract* 2009; 63(6):900–912.

31. Dhingra, R, et al. "Soft drink consumption and risk of developing cardiometabolic risk factors and the metabolic syndrome in middle-aged adults in the community." *Circulation* 2007; 116(5):480–488.

32. Abid, A, et al. "Soft drink consumption is associated with fatty liver disease independent of metabolic syndrome." *J Hepatol* 2009; 51(5):918–924.

33. Cohen, D.A, et al. "Not enough fruit and vegetables or too many cookies, salty snacks, and soft drinks?" *Public Health Rep* 2010; 125(1):88–95.

34. Davis, B. and Carpenter, C. "Proximity of fast-food restaurants to schools and adolescent obesity." *Am J Public Health* 2009; 99(3):505–510.

35. Downs, S.M, et al. "Associations among the food environment, diet quality and weight status in Cree children in Québec." *Public Health Nutr* 2009; 12(9):1504–1511.

36. Babey, S.H, et al. "Bubbling over: soda consumption and its link to obesity in California." *Policy Brief UCLA Cent Health Policy Res* 2009; (PB2009-5):1–8.

37. Bocarsly, M.E, et al. "High-fructose corn syrup causes characteristic of obesity in rats: increased body weight, body fat and triglyceride levels." *Pharmacology Biochemistry and Behavior* 2010; 97(1):101–106.

38. Elliott, S.S, et al. "Fructose, weight gain, and the insulin resistance syndrome." *Am J Clin Nutr* 2002; 76(5):911–922.

39. Bray, G.A, et al. "Consumption of high-fructose corn syrup in beverages may play a role in obesity." *Am J Clin Nutr* 2004; 79(4):537–543.

40. Swithers, S, et al. "A Role for Sweet Taste: Calorie Predictive Relations in Energy Regulation by Rats." *Behav Neurosci* 2008; 122(1):161–173.

41. Hu, F.B. and Malik, V.S. "Sugar-sweetened beverages and risk of obesity and type 2 diabetes: Epidemiologic evidence." *Physiol Behav* 2010; 100(1):47–54.

42. Jensen, T.K, et al. "Caffeine intake and semen quality in a population of 2,254 young Danish men." *Am J Epidemiol* 2010; 171(8):883–891.

43. Halldorsson, T.I, et al. "Intake of artificially sweetened soft drinks and risk of preterm delivery: a prospective cohort study of 59,334 Danish pregnant women." *Am J Clin Nutr* 2010; 92(3):626–633.

44. Ismail, A. "The cariogenicity of soft drinks in the United States." *J Am Dent Assoc* 1984; 109(2):241–245.

45. Heller, K.E, et al. "The amazing statistics and dangers of soda pop." *J Dent Res* 2002; 80(10):1949–1952.

46. Lim, S, et al. "Cariogenicity of soft drinks in low-income African-American children: a longitudinal study." *J Am Dent Assoc* 2008; 139(7):959–67.

47. Mahmood, M, et al. "Health effects of soda drinking in adolescent girls in the United Arab Emirates." *J Crit Care* 2008; 23(3):434–440.

48. Tucker, K.L, et al. "Colas, but not other carbonated beverages, are associated with low bone mineral density in older women: The Framingham Osteoporosis Study." *Am J Clin Nutr* 2006; 84(4):936–942.

49. Washington Post February 27, 2001; Page HE10.

50. Barrett-Connor, E, et al. "Coffee-associated osteoporosis offset by daily milk consumption. The Rancho Bernardo Study." *JAMA* 1994; 271(4):280–283.

51. Cummings, B.P, et al. "Dietary fructose accelerates the development of diabetes in UCD-T2DM rats: amelioration by the antioxidant, alpha-lipoic acid." *Am J Physiol Regul Integr Comp Physiol* 2010; 298(5):R1343–R1350.

52. Bolton, S, et al. "A pilot study of some physiological and psychological effects of caffeine." *Journal Orthomolecular Psychiatry* 1984; 13(1):1–7.

53. Petrie, H.J, et al. "Caffeine ingestion increases the insulin response to

an oral-glucose-tolerance test in obese men before and after weight loss." *J Clin Nut* 2009; 80(1):22–28.

54. Chen, L, et al. "Prospective study of pre-gravid sugar-sweetened beverage consumption and the risk of gestational diabetes mellitus." *Diabetes Care* 2009; 32(12): 2236–2241.

55. Ventura, E, et al. "Reduction in risk factors for type 2 diabetes mellitus in response to a low-sugar, high-fiber dietary intervention in overweight Latino adolescents." *Arch Pediatr Adolesc Med* 2009; 163(4):320–327.

56. Brown, R.J, et al. "Ingestion of diet soda before a glucose load augments glucagons like peptide-1 secretion." *Diabetes Care* 2009; 32(12):2184–2186.

57. Shuster, J, et al. "Soft drink consumption and urinary stone recurrence: a randomized prevention trial." *J Clin Epidemiol* 1992; 45(8):911–916.

58. Saldana, T.M, et al. "Carbonated beverages and chronic kidney disease." *Epidemiology* 2007; 18(4):501–506.

59. Dasgupta, J, et al. "Enhancement of rat bladder contraction by artificial sweeteners via increased extracellular Ca2+ influx." *Toxicology and Applied Pharmacology* 2006; 217(4):221–224.

Please note that the following citations correspond to their respective numbers in the inset "31 Ways Soft Drinks and Other Sweetened Beverages Can Ruin Your Health" on page 56. Some of the entries have more than one reference.

1. Vasanti, S, et al. "Intake of sugar-sweetened beverages and weight gain: a systematic review." *Am J Clin Nutr* (2006); 84(2):274–288.

Rezazadeh, A. and Rashidkhani, B."The association of general and central obesity with major dietary patterns of adult women living in Tehran, Iran." *J Nutr Sci Vitaminol* (2010); 56(2):132–138.

2. Abid, A. et al. "Soft drink consumption is associated with fatty liver disease independent of metabolic syndrome." *J Hepatol* (2009); 51(5):918–924.

3. Griffiths, R.R. and Vernotica, E. B. "Is caffeine a flavoring agent in cola soft drinks?" *Arch Fam Med* (2000); 9(8):727–734.

4. Lopez-Garcia, E, et al. "Major dietary patterns are related to plasma

concentrations of markers of inflammation and endothelial dysfunction." *Am J Clin Nutr* (2004); 80(4):1029–1035.

5. Nathias, B, et al. "Sugar-Sweetened Beverages, Weight Gain, and Incidence of Type 2 Diabetes in Young and Middle-Aged Women." *JAMA* (2004); 292(8):927–934.

6. Dhingra, R, et al. "Soft Drink Consumption and the Risk of Developing Cardiometabolic Risk Factors and the Metabolic Syndrome in Middle-Aged Adults in the Community." *Circulation* (2007); 116:457.

7. Ehlen, L.A, et al. "Acidic beverages increase the risk of in vitro tooth erosion." *Nut Research* (2008); 28(5):299–303.

8. Tucker, K.L, et al. "Colas, but not other carbonated beverages, are associated with low bone mineral density in older women: The Framingham Osteoporosis Study." *Am J Clin Nutr* (2006); 84(4):936–942.

9. Hak, A.E. and Choi, H.K. "Lifestyle and Gout." *Curr Opin Rheumatol* (2008); 20(2):179–186.

10. Bever, P.L, et al. "Fructose intake at current levels in the United States may cause gastrointestinal distress in normal adults." *J Am Diet Assoc* (2005); 105(10):1559–1566.

11. Hering-Hanit, R. and Gadoth, N. "Caffeine-induced headache in children and adolescents." *Cephalalgia* (2003); 23(5):332–335.

12. Høstmar, A.T. and Tomten, S.E. "Cola intake and serum lipids in the Oslo Health Study." *Appl Physiol Nutr Metab* (2009); 34(5):901–906.

13. Dhingra, R, et al. "Soft Drink Consumption and Risk of Developing Cardiometabolic Risk Factors and the Metabolic Syndrome in Middle-Aged Adults in the Community." *Circulation* (2007); 116(5):480–488.

14. Griffiths, R.R. and Vernotica, E. B. "Is caffeine a flavoring agent in cola soft drinks?" *Arch Fam Med* (2000); 9(8):727–734.

15. Dasgupta, J. "Enhancement of rat bladder contraction by artificial sweeteners via increased extracellular Ca2+ influx." *Toxicol Appl Pharmacol* (2006); 217(2):216–224.

16. Mueller, N.T, et al. "Soft Drink and Juice Consumption and Risk of Pancreatic Cancer: The Singapore Chinese Health Study." *Cancer Epidemiology Biomarkers & Prevention* (2010); 19(2):447.

17. Mahmood, M, et al. "Health effects of soda drinking in adolescent girls in the United Arab Emirates." *J Crit Care* (2008); 23(3):434–440.

18. Halldorsson, T.H, et al. "Intake of artificially sweetened soft drinks and risk of preterm delivery: a prospective cohort study of 59,334 Danish pregnant women." *Am J Clin Nutr* (2010); 10:3945.

Choi, H.K, et al. "Soft drinks, fructose consumption, and the risk of gout in men: prospective cohort study." *BMJ* (2008); 336(7639):309–312.

19. Davis, R.E. and Osorlo, I. "Childhood Caffeine Tic Syndrome." *Pediatrics* (1988); 101(6):e4.

20. Chen, L, et al. "Prospective Study of Pre-Gravid Sugar-Sweetened Beverage Consumption and the Risk of Gestational Diabetes Mellitus." *Diabetes Care* (2009); 32(12):2236.

21. Packer, C.D. "Chronic hypokalemia due to excessive cola consumption: a case report." *Cases J* (2008); 1(1):32.

22. "Eating High Levels of Fructose Impairs Memory in Rats." www.sciencedaily.com

23. Kirdpon, W, et al. "Soft drink consumption and urinary stone." *J Clin Epidem* (1992); 45:911–916.

24. Jensen, T.K, et al. "Caffeine Intake and Semen Quality in a Population of 2,554 Young Danish Men." *Am J Epidem* (2010); 171(8):883–891.

25. Luebbe, A.M. and Bell, D.J. "Mountain Dew or mountain don't?: a pilot investigation of caffeine use parameters and relations to depression and anxiety symptoms in 5th- and 10th-grade students." *J Sch Health* (2009); 79(8):380–387.

26. Elliott, J.O, et al. "Exercise, diet, health behaviors, and risk factors among persons with epilepsy based on the California Health Interview Survey, 2005." *Epilepsy Behav* (2008); 13(2):307–315.

27. Vandeloo, M.J, et al. "Effects of lifestyle on the onset of puberty as determinant for breast cancer." *Euro J Cancer Prevent* (2007); 16(1):17–25.

28. Nguyen, S. et al. "Sugar-sweetened beverages, serum uric acid, and blood pressure in adolescents." *J Pediatr* (2000); 154(6):807–813.

29. Hattah, F.N, et al. "Dental discoloration: an overview." *J Esthet Dent* (1999); 11(6):291–310.

30. Dasgupta, J, et al. "Enhancement of rat bladder contraction by artificial sweeteners via increased extracellular Ca2+ influx." *Toxicology and Applied Pharmacology* (2006): 217(4):221–224.

Mallath, M.K. "Carbonated soft drink consumption and risk of esophageal adenocarcinoma." *J Natl Cancer Inst* (2006); 98(9):644–645.

31. "Drinking Soda Linked To Gullet Cancer Rise." www.newscientist.com

Chapter 6

1. Adams, M. *The Five Soft Drink Monsters*. Toledo, OH: Truth Publishing, LLC, 2005.

2. Griffiths, R.R, et al. "Is caffeine a flavoring agent in cola soft drinks?" *Arch Fam Med* 2000; 9:727–734.

3. Avena, N.N, et al. "Evidence for sugar addiction: behavioral and neurochemical effects of intermittent, excessive sugar intake." *Neurosci Biobehav Rev* 2008; 32(1):20–39.

4. Roberts, H.J. "Aspartame (NutraSweet) Addiction." *Townsend Letter for Doctors & Patients* 2000; 198:52–57.

5. Selye, H. *The Stress of Life*. New York: McGraw-Hill, 1954.

6. www.kaysheppard.com

Chapter 7

1. Greenberg, B.S. "A portrait of food and drink in commercial TV series." *Health Commun* 2009; 24(4):295–303.

2. "Family Doctors Sign Educational Deal with Coca-Cola." www.npr.org

3. "Aspartame has been renamed and is now being marketed as a natural sweetener." www.naturalnews.com

Chapter 8

1. "Statement Regarding Release of the Evaluation of School Beverage Guidelines." www.rwjf.org

2. Block, J.P, et al. "Point-of-Purchase Price and Education Intervention to Reduce Consumption of Sugary Soft Drinks." *Am J Public Health* 2010; 100(8):1427–1433.

3. Brownell, K.D, et al. "The Public Health and Economic Benefits of Taxing Sugar- Sweetened Beverages." *N E J Med* 2009; 361(16):1599–1605.

About the Authors

Nancy Appleton earned her BS in clinical nutrition from UCLA and her Ph.D. in health services from Walden University. She graduated with honors from Walden University with her award-winning dissertation, *An Alternative to the Germ Theory*. She has retired from her private practice and lives in San Diego, but continues to research and write about nutrition and health issues. She has appeared on radio, TV, and Internet broadcasts. In addition to *Killer Colas*, she has written several books on nutrition and health: *Suicide by Sugar, Stopping Inflammation, Healthy Bones, Lick the Sugar Habit, Lick the Sugar Habit Sugar Counter*, and *Curse of Louis Pasteur*. You can contact Nancy at **nancyappletonbooks@yahoo.com** or visit her website at **www.nancyappleton.com**

G.N. Jacobs (Greg to his friends) is a reporter, novelist, essayist, and many other job titles that involve words on paper. He is proud of his first novel *Blood & Ink* and his subsequent short story collection *The Beast that Almost Ate Los Angeles*. His work with Dr. Appleton started out as a client and blossomed from there. He also co-wrote *Suicide by Sugar* with Dr. Appleton. He lives in Los Angeles where he writes several blogs, including one about *Star Trek*. Presently, he's hard at work on several new books.

Index

Order Forms

AUDIO CDS

Lick the Sugar Habit—An introduction to the book of the same name, this disk provides detailed explanations of the body chemistry principle, mineral relationships, enzyme function, and causes of infectious and degenerative disease. (1 hour)

Allergies—What are food allergies? What causes them? How can they be eliminated? Learn how foods to which you have allergic reactions can be reintroduced to your diet. The similar role of environmental allergies is also discussed. (1 hour)

Osteoporosis—Although you may be getting enough calcium in your diet, if you're out of homeostasis, this mineral can't be absorbed properly. This disk explains how to look for symptoms of calcium deficiency and how to test for susceptibility to osteoporosis. (1 hour)

Women/Obesity—A combined disk with two sections starting with the latest information concerning pre-menstrual syndrome, Candida (yeast) infections, menstruation, menopause, and post-menopause problems. The second section relates information about the latest research on the relationship of allergies, addictions, and cravings to obesity. (1 hour)

Children—This disk begins with prenatal nutrition and continues with information about food allergies and eating problems in children. Ideas for convincing children of all ages to eat nutritious foods fill out the end of the tape. (1 hour)

Food Preparation—This disk answers some important questions. Where can I shop for the most nutritious foods? How should I prepare food to preserve health and maintain my family's and mine body chemistry? What about additives, irradiation, pesticides, and fungicides? (1 hour)

The Body Monitor—How do you test for homeostasis with urine and saliva testing? What are the common causes for being out of homeostasis? How do you regain homeostasis once you are out? This disk answers these questions. (45 minutes)

Diet and the Immune System—This disk presents an overview of the whole Body Chemistry Principle in this recording made live in 1996. Dr. Appleton explains many things and answers questions from the audience. (78 minutes)

Additional Information—Dr. Appleton naturally found more information to present after recording the disks above. This CD covers a wide variety of topics left unsaid on other recordings. (1 hour)

AUDIO CD ORDER FORM

Name: _____

Address: _____ Apt. _____

City: _____

State: _____ Zip: _____

List CD Titles:

1. _____   5. _____

2. _____   6. _____

3. _____   7. _____

4. _____   8. _____

Price List (U.S. Currency)

Quantity	Price	Shipping
1 CD	$ 8.00	$2.50
Additional CDs	$ 8.00 each	$ .50 each
All 9 CDs	$50.00	$6.00

*California residents must include local sales tax or 9.75%.

Foreign Orders: Canadian residents may use this form, but residents of other countries are requested to use our online ordering system at (www.nancy appleton.com) to shorten response time and properly deal with the varying postage costs for foreign countries. Canadian residents must send an International Money Order in U.S. Funds, as personal checks may not clear.

To order: Please send a check or money order made out to Nancy Appleton, PhD with a copy of this form to:
Nancy Appleton Books
5950 Buckingham Parkway
Culver City, CA 90230

You can also contact Nancy Appleton at
nancyappletonbooks@yahoo.com
or visit her website at www.nancyappleton.com.

BODY MONITOR TEST KIT

This kit contains testing materials to determine if your body is in homeostasis, or balance. Included are a bottle of solution for 250 urine tests, two test tubes, pipe cleaner, an eyedropper, a roll of pH paper and the 28-page instruction booklet *How to Monitor Your Basic Health*. The instructions explain how to test your urine for calcium and properly read the results. The instructions also include information on using the pH paper to test the acidity/alkalinity of both urine and saliva. Information on how to relate these results to your health, along with suggestions for the many things you can do to improve your health, are also presented—especially how the kit may be used to test for allergies. Nancy Appleton Books also adds, at no extra charge, two audio CDs: "Body Monitor" and "Diet and the Immune System" in order to provide additional understanding of the Body Chemistry Principle.

Name: _____

Address: _____ Apt. _____

City:_____

State: _____ Zip: _____

Price List (U.S. Currency)

Quantity	Price	Shipping
1 Kit	$33.00	$8.00

California residents must include local sales tax or 9.75%.

Foreign Orders: Canadian residents may use this form, but residents of other countries are requested to use our online ordering system at (www.nancyappleton.com) to shorten response time and properly deal with the varying postage costs for foreign countries. Canadian residents must send an International Money Order in U.S. Funds, as personal checks may not clear.

To order: Please send a check or money order made out to Nancy Appleton, PhD with a copy of this form to:
Nancy Appleton Books
5950 Buckingham Parkway
Culver City, CA 90230

You can also contact Nancy Appleton at
nancyappletonbooks@yahoo.com
or visit her website at www.nancyappleton.com.

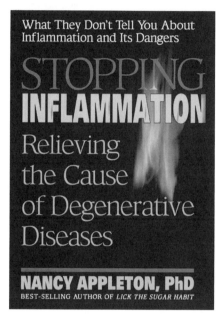

What They Don't Tell You About Inflammation and Its Dangers

STOPPING INFLAMMATION
Relieving the Cause of Degenerative Diseases
Nancy Appleton, PhD

Most of us think of inflammation as a symptom associated with an infection or injury. Dr. Nancy Appleton, however, has discovered that it might be more than just a simple reaction to a health disorder. When the body's tissues are disturbed in some manner, a series of complex reactions takes place, resulting in inflammation. In most cases, when the disorder stops, the tissue returns to its normal healthy state. Sometimes, though, the tissue remains chronically inflamed. Dr. Appleton's research demonstrates that this condition might be more harmful than ever suspected.

Drawing on the latest medical research, *Stopping Inflammation* begins with a full explanation of inflammation and its causes. It then looks at inflammation's role in various health disorders, from obesity to cancer. Finally, the book provides a number of nondrug treatments aimed not at controlling the problem, but at removing its cause. Here are safe and credible solutions for restoring good health.

$14.95 • 224 pages • 6 x 9-inch quality paperback • ISBN 978-0-7570-0418-2

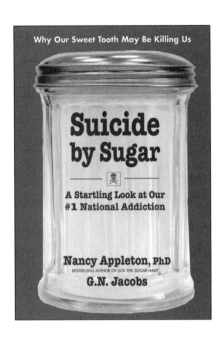

Why Our Sweet Tooth May Be Killing Us

Suicide by Sugar

☠

A Startling Look at Our
#1 National Addiction

Nancy Appleton, PhD
BESTSELLING AUTHOR OF LICK THE SUGAR HABIT

G.N. Jacobs

SUICIDE BY SUGAR

A Startling Look at Our #1 National Addiction

Nancy Appleton, PhD
and G.N. Jacobs

It is a dangerous, addictive white powder that can be found in abundance throughout this country. It is not illegal. In fact, it is available in or near playgrounds, schools, workplaces, homes, and vacation spots. It is in practically everything we eat and drink, and, once we're hooked on it, the cravings can be overwhelming. This white substance of abuse is sugar. Once associated only with cavities and simple weight gain, it is now linked to a host of devastating health conditions including cancer, epilepsy, dementia, hypoglycemia, obesity, and more. In this book, sugar addiction expert Dr. Nancy Appleton and health writer G.N. Jacobs not only expose the exorbitant levels of sugar we ingest, but also document the connection between our current health crisis and our sweet tooth.

Suicide by Sugar begins with the story of Dr. Appleton's battle with her own sugar addiction. Next, the authors examine all the frightening (and unknown) things that can go wrong when people consume too much sugar—from increased susceptibility to disease to imbalanced body chemistry. They go on to discuss the various ways scientists measure sugar's impact on blood glucose, and explain why these statistics cannot be solely relied on when choosing foods. The authors provide shocking information about the amount of sugar found in many popular foods and beverages, and an in-depth discussion of the ailments now associated with excessive sugar consumption. Finally, Dr. Appleton's easy-to-follow, effective lifestyle plan—complete with recipes—guides you in eliminating sugar from your life.

As children, we fall under the spell of ads that lure us to indulge in all things sweet. Is it any wonder that as adults, so few of us can see the dark side of sugar? *Suicide by Sugar* shines a bright light on our nation's addiction and helps us begin the journey toward health.

$15.95 • 192 pages • 6 x 9-inch paperback • ISBN 978-0-7570-0306-6

What You Must Know About Vitamins, Minerals, Herbs & More
Choosing the Nutrients That Are Right for You
Pamela Wartian Smith, MD, MPH

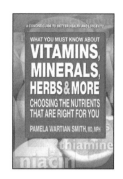

Almost 75 percent of health and longevity is based on lifestyle, environment, and nutrition. Yet even if you follow a healthful diet, you probably don't get all the nutrients you need to prevent disease. In this book, Dr. Pamela Smith explains how you can maintain health through the use of nutrients.

Part One of this easy-to-use guide discusses the individual nutrients necessary for good health. Part Two offers personalized nutritional programs for people with a wide variety of health concerns. People without prior medical problems can look to Part Three for their supplementation plans. Whether you want to maintain good health or you are trying to overcome a medical condition, *What You Must Know About Vitamins, Minerals, Herbs & More* can help you make the best choices for the health and well-being of you and your family.

$15.95 US • 448 pages • 6 x 9-inch quality paperback • ISBN 978-0-7570-0233-5

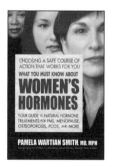

What You Must Know About Women's Hormones
Your Guide to Natural Hormone Treatments for PMS, Menopause, Osteoporosis, PCOS, and More
Pamela Wartian Smith, MD, MPH

Hormonal imbalances can occur at any age and for a variety of reasons. While most related problems are associated with menopause, fluctuating hormonal levels can also cause a variety of other conditions. *What You Must Know About Women's Hormones* is a guide to the treatment of hormonal irregularities without the health risks associated with standard hormone replacement therapy.

Part I of this book describes the body's own hormones, looking at their functions and the problems that can occur if they are not at optimal levels. Part II focuses on the most common problems that arise from hormonal imbalances, such as PMS and endometriosis. Part III details hormone replacement therapy, focusing on the difference between natural and synthetic treatments. *What You Must Know About Women's Hormones* can make a profound difference in your life.

$17.95 US • 256 pages • 6 x 9-inch quality paperback • ISBN 978-0-7570-0307-3

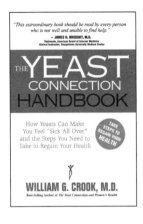

THE YEAST CONNECTION HANDBOOK

How Yeasts Can Make You Feel "Sick All Over" and the Steps You Need to Take to Regain Your Health

William G. Crook, MD

The Yeast Connection Handbook is a great resource for anyone who wants to learn about yeast-related problems. The book not only discusses a wide range of health issues, from fatigue to sexual dysfunction, but also addresses a range of sufferers, including men, women, and children. Most important, it offers a step-by-step program that effectively relieves disorders through dietary and lifestyle changes, nutritional supplements, and medication.

$15.95 US • 288 pages • 6 x 9-inch quality paperback • ISBN 978-0-7570-0060-7

THE YEAST CONNECTION COOKBOOK

A Guide to Good Nutrition, Better Health and Weight Management

William G. Crook, MD, and Marjorie Hurt Jones, RN

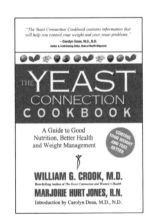

What can you eat if you have a yeast-related problem? *The Yeast Connection Cookbook* provides general information on the effects that some common foods can have on yeast sufferers, and key instructions for detecting the specific foods to which you are particularly sensitive or allergic. The authors then present over 225 recipes—for breads, soups, entrées, desserts, and more—that eliminate most common food allergens while providing a diet that is healthful and satisfying.

$15.95 US • 384 pages • 6 x 9-inch quality paperback • ISBN 978-0-7570-0059-1

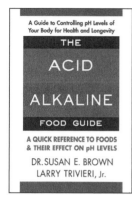

THE ACID-ALKALINE FOOD GUIDE
A Quick Reference to Foods & Their Effect on pH Levels
Dr. Susan E. Brown and Larry Trivieri, Jr.

In the last few years, researchers around the world have reported the importance of acid-alkaline balance to good health. While thousands of people are trying to balance their body's pH level, until now, they have had to rely on guides containing only a small number of foods. *The Acid-Alkaline Food Guide* is a complete resource for people who want to widen their food choices.

The book begins by explaining how the acid-alkaline environment of the body is influenced by foods. It then presents a list of thousands of foods—single foods, combination foods, and even fast foods—and their acid-alkaline effects. *The Acid-Alkaline Food Guide* will quickly become the resource you turn to at home, in restaurants, and whenever you want to select a food that can help you reach your health and dietary goals.

$7.95 • 208 pages • 4 x 7-inch mass paperback • ISBN 978-0-7570-0280-9

GLYCEMIC INDEX FOOD GUIDE
For Weight Loss, Cardiovascular Health, Diabetic Management, and Maximum Energy
Dr. Shari Lieberman

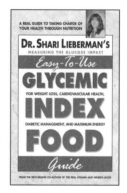

By indicating how quickly a given food triggers a rise in blood sugar, the glycemic index (GI) enables you to choose foods that can help you manage various conditions and improve your overall health. Designed as an easy-to-use guide to the glycemic index, this book first answers commonly asked questions, to ensure that you truly understand the GI and know how to use it. It then provides both the glycemic index and the glycemic load for hundreds of foods and beverages.

$7.95 • 160 pages • 4 x 7-inch mass paperback • ISBN 978-0-7570-0245-8

**For more information about our books,
visit our website at www.squareonepublishers.com**

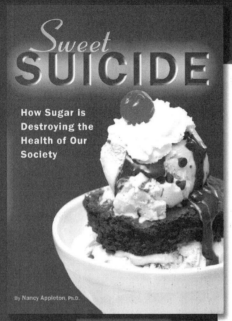